# DEAFNESS AND HEARING LOSS

## The Essential Guide

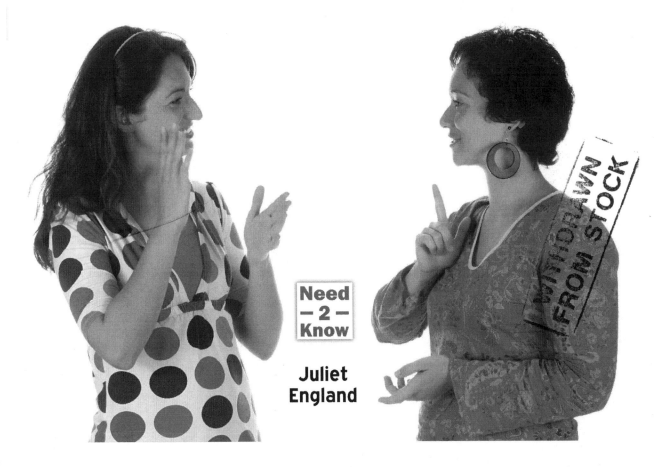

**Need — 2 — Know**

**Juliet England**

First published in Great Britain in 2010 by
**Need2Know**
Remus House
Coltsfoot Drive
Peterborough
PE2 9JX
Telephone 01733 898103
Fax 01733 313524
www.need2knowbooks.co.uk

Need2Know is an imprint of Forward Press Ltd.
www.forwardpress.co.uk
All Rights Reserved
© Juliet England 2010
SB ISBN 978-1-86144-078-5
Cover photograph: Stockxpert

# Contents

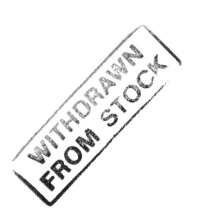

# Introduction

Every day in the UK, four deaf babies are born and there are 35,000 deaf children in the UK at any one time. Many others will go on to develop a hearing loss at some point in their lives. In all, there are almost nine million people in the UK with a hearing problem of some kind – that's 1 in 7.

And, of course, an even greater number of people are affected in some way – colleagues, parents, partners and family members. Almost all of us will come into contact with a deaf or hard of hearing person at some point in our lives.

There are several different kinds of hearing loss, and deafness does not have a single cause. Various factors – environmental, genetic, injuries and disease – can all come into play. Hearing loss should not just be associated with old age, although nearly three quarters of those over 70 will have some kind of hearing difficulty, and in the UK there are more than half a million people aged 60 or over who are severely or profoundly deaf.

In spite of the sterling work of RNID, the National Deaf Children's Society (NDCS) and others, and despite the Disability Discrimination Act (DDA), too many deaf and hard of hearing people still face barriers to success and come across prejudice in their daily lives. Every deaf person who fails to reach their full potential is one too many.

Discrimination can take many forms – from an employer who doesn't give their hard of hearing colleague the promotion they deserve, to a college student not getting the support they need. It can be direct or indirect. Sometimes, just a simple refusal to repeat something to someone with a hearing difficulty can be enough to make them feel excluded, especially if it's an apparently hilarious joke which everyone else seems to be enjoying.

Losing your hearing, or even just some of it, can be a distressing experience, as can the shock of an initial diagnosis. Whether you're a fashion-conscious teenager suddenly told you will have to wear a hearing aid for the rest of your life or a parent with a new baby newly diagnosed with a hearing problem, it can be a bewildering and upsetting time.

There are various lingering myths surrounding deafness and hearing problems. Incredibly, the association with deafness and a lack of intelligence persists. And there are other misconceptions. Too many people, for example, still think that the best way of making a deaf or hard of hearing person understand is to shout at them. In fact, shouting just distorts the sound and is one of the worst things you can do.

Another common misunderstanding is that all deaf or hard of hearing people share the same degree and type of hearing loss, yet nothing could be further from the truth. There is a huge difference between being deaf and having a mild hearing loss, for example.

Depending on its severity, hearing loss is classed as mild, moderate, moderately severe, severe or profound. Severity often depends to an extent on the age of onset of the problem. Two people with the same degree of hearing loss may experience it very differently depending on how old they were when it began.

Along with these categorisations, there are three main types of hearing loss – conductive (where there are problems with sound passing through the inner or outer ear), sensorineural (where the source of the problem is the cochlea or hearing nerve) or mixed hearing loss, which is a combination of both.

In this guide, we'll look at these categories in more detail and discuss deafness and hearing loss at every stage of life. We'll also consider tinnitus – the persistent buzzing, hissing or booming sound heard in the absence of any environmental explanation – which for many is every bit as challenging as a hearing loss or difficulty. Many people with a hearing loss also experience tinnitus.

We'll look at the different communications tools on the market – and how they can help. There have, of course, been great technological strides in recent years, making it easier than ever for deaf people to communicate, including email, improved phones, digital hearing aids and other devices.

There are many issues such as cochlear implants and 'glue ear' which we'll consider as well.

This book is for those who have hearing problems, but also parents, teachers, employers and carers.

Despite the problems it can pose, for many people, deafness is a positive aspect of their identity and a huge source of pride. Many deaf people do reach their potential and lead full and richly rewarding lives. The aim of this guide is to give you the information and access to resources you need, so that you can become one of them, or help someone else to fulfil their potential.

N.B. People can be hearing impaired, deaf, deaf and deafened. When I use the term deaf, hard of hearing or hearing impaired in this book, I use it to embrace all kinds of hearing loss, temporary and permanent.

## Acknowledgements

I am grateful to the many people who gave their help when I was researching and putting together this book. I thank them here in no particular order.

Thanks to Dr Lindsay Peer for her gracious help in allowing me to refer to her book, *Glue Ear: An Essential Guide for Teachers, Parents and Health Professionals* (David Fulton Publishers, 2005), for the chapter I have written about glue ear.

I am especially grateful to the British Tinnitus Association, the National Deaf Children's Society (NDCS) and RNID for giving me guidance and a great deal of information throughout, and to the National Institution of Clinical Evidence (NICE) and Deafness Research UK.

Lisa Waite, hearing therapist at the Royal Berkshire Hospital's audiology department, was another invaluable source of information.

My thanks also to Ruth Edwards and staff and pupils at Henry Beaufort School, Winchester, for allowing me to visit the deaf unit there and to Dr Lesley Black at the University of Winchester for her comments about deafness in higher education.

I am indebted as well to Carol May for her guidance on the education chapter and to Hampshire County Council's education department for their assistance with the same section.

Various interviewees gave me their time very generously and I could not have written this book without their help. They include Phil Creighton, Lisa Whiting, Michael Lawson and Helen Akers. Lisa Dillon and Sam Forrester spoke to me about their experiences as parents of deaf children with great openness and emotional depth.

Nigel Sinfield at Virgin Media was painstaking in his help with the section on subtitling, and Malcolm Gregory at the law firm Withy King was equally meticulous in reviewing the chapter on deafness and employment.

The help of all these people has been invaluable. Finally, my thanks to Graham Wilks, quite possibly the world's fussiest proofreader.

## Disclaimer

This book is intended to give information about deafness and hearing loss in general terms only. It should not be used in place of professional medical advice but can be used alongside such advice. Anyone with concerns about either their own or someone else's hearing should go to their GP in the first instance.

Interviewees who appear in the book have had their names changed where requested.

This publication is entirely independent and is not endorsed in any way by any of the organisations mentioned in the book.

# Chapter One

## Definitions

Let's start with some basic definitions and facts and figures. Terms such as 'hearing loss', 'hard of hearing' and 'deaf' are bandied around so commonly, it can be easy to lose sight of what they really mean.

- Deaf people are not just those who can't hear anything. In fact, the term is used very generally to refer to people with all kinds of hearing loss, including the severely and profoundly deaf and those who were born deaf.

- Hard of hearing people are those with a mild to severe hearing loss. Often, this term is used to describe a hearing loss which has been gradual and developed over a period of time.

- Deafened people are those who were usually able to hear when they were born, but, after they learned to speak, they became severely or profoundly deaf.

## Some basic facts and figures

RNID says there are around nine million deaf or hard of hearing people in the UK today. Most have developed a hearing loss over time, and, as the population ages, the number of people who struggle to hear is increasing all the time. The most common statistic you will hear is that 1 in 7 will have a hearing problem of some kind at some point in their lives.

By comparison, some 2% of young adults are deaf or hard of hearing and around 20,000 children under the age of 15 are moderately to profoundly deaf. Not to mention the fact that many more children have temporary hearing problems when they are very young.

According to the Institute of Hearing Research Statistics, five million people, or more than 11% of the total population, have a mild hearing loss; 2.2 million, or just under 5% of the general population, are moderately deaf; and 300,000 are severely or profoundly deaf.

RNID reports the following statistics:

- There are nearly 2.5 million deaf and hard of hearing people in the UK aged between 16 and 60.

- Some 688,000 are severely or profoundly deaf.

# Degrees of deafness

'There are nearly 2.5 million deaf and hard of hearing people in the UK aged between 16 and 60.'

RNID

Volume of sound is measured in units called decibels and there are various frequencies of sound, with tones ranging from high to low. To hear properly, we need to take in the full spectrum of tonal differences. We need depth of sound as well as volume.

Most of the useful sounds we need to understand speech are to be found in consonants, which are to be found in the middle and high tones.

- Someone with a mild hearing loss can hear at 20-40 decibels. They will usually be able to hold conversations with one other person if the room is not noisy. However, they may well experience difficulties when more than one other person is talking at the same time, or if there is a lot of background noise. A mild hearing loss is one which falls just outside the normal range of hearing.

- A person who has a moderate hearing loss may struggle to hear even if the room is relatively quiet or when speaking one-to-one. A moderate loss generally means you can hear at between 41-70 decibels.

- Someone with a severe hearing loss may appear to ignore communication completely. However, the loss means they can only hear at between 71-95 decibels. They may be able to hear environmental sounds and some vowels, but hearing and distinguishing consonants may be extremely difficult or even impossible.

■ A profound hearing loss means that other forms of communication will be necessary and it will not be enough to rely on a hearing aid or the person's own hearing. This is usually a loss at above 95 decibels.

# Types of deafness

Broadly speaking, deafness can be divided into three main categories.

■ Conductive deafness occurs when sound is not conducted properly through the outer ear, middle ear, or both. Essentially, this means that while the inner ear (or cochlea) may be functioning normally, the sounds are not being transmitted to it properly. This type of difficulty is, more often than not, a mild to moderate impairment since the inner ear can still detect sound, although more severe impairments do occur.

■ Sensorineural hearing loss is caused by insensitivity of the inner ear, the cochlea, or because the auditory nervous system (hearing nerve) is not functioning as it should. With this kind of loss, the potential for a more serious loss, up to and including total deafness, can be greater.

■ Mixed hearing loss involves the inner and outer or middle ears.

Some people may also experience hyperacusis – or an unusual sensitivity to sounds, meaning that even ordinary sounds can seem uncomfortably loud.

# Causes of deafness

There are various reasons why someone may not be able to hear properly:

■ Ageing is the single most common factor (age-related deafness is called presbyacusis) but of course there are other causes of deafness and hearing loss. More than half (55%) of people aged 60 or older are deaf or hard of hearing. This rises to 90% of those aged over 80. Typically, presbycusis causes deterioration of the higher frequencies, so that high-pitched sounds like consonants are not heard so well and speech starts to become indistinct or muffled.

- Hereditary – some hearing problems can be inherited. This includes genetic conditions such as otosclerosis, a middle ear condition causing a slow hearing loss. It can be treated with hearing aids and, sometimes, surgery.

- Tympanosclerosis is a condition in which there is calcification of tissue in the middle ear.

- Diseases of the ear – middle ear infections and perforated eardrums can be responsible for causing a hearing loss.

- Noise exposure can also affect some people's hearing. This can be work-related. For example, people in the construction industry are especially vulnerable and should take particular care to protect their ears and their hearing. Dentists' hearing can also sometimes be affected by the noise of drilling.

- Some cancer treatments have also been found to affect the patient's hearing. This is called ototoxicity and it occurs when a toxin damages the cochlea or auditory nerve. Potentially ototoxic drugs include some antibiotics and some platinum-based agents used in chemotherapy. This kind of hearing loss is generally sensorineural and may be either temporary (and treatable) or irreversible and permanent.

- Loss of hair cells in the inner ear, or cochlea. This is a natural process and we all tend to start to lose these 100,000 cells as we grow older, but if this is accelerated, early onset hearing loss will result.

- Traumas such as head injuries can also cause sensorineural hearing loss.

## How the ear works

Your ear is a marvel of engineering! It is essentially divided into three parts – outer, middle and inner ear. The middle ear, an air-filled cavity, is connected to the nose and throat via the Eustachian tube.

You hear when sound waves come into the ear and travel down the ear canal to the eardrum. The eardrum, also called the tympanic membrane, is a thin barrier between the outer and middle ears and when sound waves reach it, the

'Your ear is a marvel of engineering! It is essentially divided into three parts – outer, middle and inner ear. The middle ear, an air-filled cavity, is connected to the nose and throat via the Eustachian tube.'

eardrum starts to move. This then causes three tiny bones, or ossicles, located behind the eardrum to vibrate. (To give them their technical names, these bones are called the malleus, the stapes and the incus.)

The smallest of the three bones, the stapes, transmits sound into a part of the inner ear called the cochlea – a chamber filled with fluid which looks a bit like a snail shell. The cochlea is full of thousands of minuscule hair cells which sense the sound vibrations and convert them into electrical nerve signals. The auditory nerve passes this information on to your brain, which in turn converts these signals into what we experience as sound.

As well as the cochlea, the inner ear also contains the vestibular system – a fluid-filled area with three small sections. The fluid moves when you turn your head, causing electrical signals to be sent to your brain. Your brain then uses the information to help you keep your balance.

# Summing Up

- People can be deaf, hard of hearing or deafened.

- 1 in 7 of us will develop some kind of hearing problem at some point in our lives.

- Britain's population of deaf and hard of hearing people is around nine million.

- Deafness can be moderate, mild, severe or profound.

- Deafness can also be conductive, sensorineural or mixed.

- Hearing loss has a wide range of causes, from noise exposure to hereditary factors and ageing.

- The ear is a complex and finely balanced organ made up of three sections.

# Chapter Two

# Hearing Loss in Childhood

Permanent deafness in childhood is much rarer than it is in adulthood, and it brings with it a completely different set of issues and needs. For that reason, the professionals working with deaf children use different strategies when working with them as a separate group.

One of the distinctive aspects of hearing difficulties in childhood is that adults have already fully developed language skills, and so they do not have to take on new ideas and concepts by listening as children do, for example at school. Equally, the adult brain is able to fill in gaps where speech hasn't been completely heard, and in doing so can make sense of what is being heard. Children have not yet acquired this ability.

So deafness in childhood can affect speech and language development. It can also have an impact on a child's social and educational development and sometimes their motor development as well.

Deafness in childhood covers the whole spectrum of frequencies and can range from just below the normal range of hearing (mild deafness) right the way through to moderate, severe, profound and total deafness.

As with adults, hearing aids and cochlear implants can be used to bring hearing levels up so that all speech frequencies can be heard, allowing the child's spoken language to develop.

'For children, hearing aids and cochlear implants can be used to bring hearing levels up so that all speech frequencies can be heard, allowing the child's spoken language to develop.'

## Statistics on deafness in childhood

Deafness in childhood may be less common than in adulthood, but 15 children are born in England each week with a permanent hearing impairment. Put differently, four babies are born deaf every single day.

Research shows that about 3.47 per 1,000 children at school entry age will have a permanent hearing loss (see Bamford et al., 2007). Around half of all permanently deaf children are born deaf, the other 50% become deaf during childhood (see Fortnum et al., 2001).

# Causes of deafness in childhood

## Temporary deafness

■ Glue ear is by far the commonest cause of deafness in childhood and we will deal with this subject more fully in chapter 3. In the majority of cases, it is a temporary condition – by the time they are eight years old, most children will have grown out of it. At any one time, 20% of 1-3-year-olds will have glue ear.

■ Meningitis can cause hearing loss in various ways. Among the most common are the spreading of the infection into the inner ear, damaging the cochlea and causing inflammation of the auditory nerve. Parents are urged to ensure that all children who have had meningitis attend a hearing test within four weeks of being discharged from hospital. Meningitis can also cause permanent deafness. Indeed, according to Deafness Research UK, deafness is the most common of all forms of permanent damage following this disease and can affect up to 10% of all those who recover from it. Bacterial meningitis accounts for around 6% of all hearing impairment in children. Meningitis can also leave children with tinnitus.

## Permanent deafness

A genetic factor is behind half of all cases of permanent deafness in children.

The causes of the other half include:

■ Congenital infection (e.g. CMV, syphilis).

■ Oxygen deprivation at birth.

■ Being born extremely prematurely.

- Severe jaundice, among other childhood illnesses.
- Oxotoxic medication (as described in chapter 1) such as gentamycin or some kinds of chemotherapy.

# Screening in childhood and detecting problems

Since March 2006, parents in England have been offered the opportunity to have their newborn baby's hearing screened shortly after birth through the NHS Newborn Hearing Screening Programme. Most children also have their hearing tested when they start school. However, in practice, in a tenth of all areas in the UK, school entry screening is no longer provided.

## Newborn hearing screening

All newborn babies need to be screened as early as possible to prevent any delays with language development which might otherwise result. A deaf child can develop language at the same rate as their hearing peers providing that deafness is identified by the time they're six months old and an early programme of intervention and support is in place.

Around 90% of deaf babies are born into families who have no previous history or experience of hearing problems (see Rawlings and Jensema, 1977). Some babies with hearing loss will respond to some sounds, so you may not even be aware there is a problem – this shows just how important screening is to identify difficulties.

There are two quick and simple screening tests, neither of which will cause any harm or discomfort. They can be done while the baby is asleep or settled and a parent can stay with their baby at all times. You may find it's easier to do the test if the baby is asleep, so you may want to try and do a feed beforehand and make your baby comfortable. Depending on the local arrangements in your area, the tests are carried out either at home, in a hospital or at a local GP surgery or health clinic, and will be done by a health visitor or a trained hearing screener.

The results are given straightaway and you can discuss any questions or concerns with your hospital, GP or health visitor at the same time.

'All newborn babies need to be screened as early as possible to prevent any delays with language development.'

## Automated otoacoustic emission screening test

An automated otoacoustic emission (AOAE) only takes a few minutes. A small soft-tipped earpiece is placed in the outer part of your baby's ear, which sends sounds down the ear. The cochlea in the inner ear should produce an echo as it receives the sound. The screening equipment can pick up this reaction.

Sometimes, for various reasons, a second test has to be done, but this doesn't necessarily mean your baby has a hearing loss. The test may be a repeat of the first one, or it could be one of the following tests.

## Automated auditory brainstem response screening test

An automated auditory brainstem response (AABR) test can take up to half an hour to complete. Three small sensors will be placed on your baby's head and neck and soft headphones placed over their ears. Some clicking sounds will be played and the screening equipment can show how well your baby's ears respond to sound.

Most babies have a clear response following a second screening test, but it is still recommended that you have it done. If the test does show a clear response in both of your baby's ears, they are unlikely to have any hearing loss. However, this does not necessarily mean a loss may not develop later in childhood, and your child's hearing can be tested at any time, so discuss any concerns with your GP or health visitor.

Parents are given checklists to help monitor their child's development, as a child can develop hearing problems at any age, and for a number of reasons.

If the second test gives cause for concern, you will be referred to a local audiology department which will carry out further tests to create a fuller picture about your child's hearing. Even at this stage, you should still not necessarily assume that your child has a hearing loss. Although it is possible that your baby may have a hearing problem, only about 1 in 25 infants whose second test doesn't show clear responses may turn out to have a hearing loss in one or both ears.

'It's important to remember that by identifying a problem at an early stage, you give yourself the best possible chance of getting the advice, information and support you and your baby need from the outset.'

It's important to remember that by identifying a problem at an early stage, you give yourself the best possible chance of getting the advice, information and support you and your baby need from the outset.

You can find more information about hearing testing and screening from your midwife, GP, health visitor or local audiology department.

The government stresses that action should always be taken where parents express concern about their child's hearing. Parents, health visitors, teachers, GPs and others must be vigilant in referring a child for testing if they suspect a hearing loss between screening at birth and school entry.

## Signs to watch for in older children

Potential indicators of hearing problems include:

- Delayed speech development.
- A child failing to respond when they are called.
- Difficulty identifying the direction a particular sound comes from.
- Constantly needing the TV on louder than other family members.
- Behavioural changes, including increased tiredness and/or frustration.
- Poor concentration and a preference for solitary playing.
- Changes in educational progress.
- Frequent ear infections.

## What can I do to protect my child's hearing?

If your child has noisy toys, limit the amount of time spent playing with them and try to stop them from holding them too close to their ears.

If children often participate in noisy leisure activities then hearing protection is recommended. You can buy ear muffs from manufacturers such as Peltor.

They can cost as little as £15, so ear muffs are a relatively affordable form of ear protection.

# Young people and ear protection from loud music

## Live music and nightclubs

Teenagers (as well as adults) who regularly go to nightclubs should try not to dance directly in front of a speaker if at all possible. It's also good advice to have a 15-20 minute break once an hour away from the dance floor in a quieter area.

Foam ear plugs are also widely available. Even basic yellow foam earplugs reduce the overall level of noise. These cheap earplugs are made as one-size-fits-all, but, if you are willing to pay more, they can be custom-made. These kinds of tailor-made ear plugs are popular with musicians, who have to wear them for extended periods.

## Recorded music

Some MP3 players have noise-limiting software to keep the volume of music within safe levels. If your MP3 player doesn't come with this software already, it can sometimes be downloaded after purchase.

Children should be encouraged to take frequent breaks from wearing headphones. Set the volume of the MP3 player to a reasonable level and try not to turn it up when background noise levels rise, as this can take total noise levels above what is considered safe. Good quality noise-cancelling headphones can be purchased that help to reduce the effects of background noise, allowing the listener to keep the music at a lower level, reducing the risk of damaging their ears.

For children or young people who wear hearing aids, the aids can be linked directly to the music player so that they benefit from the hearing aids' personal amplification programme.

'Some MP3 players have noise-limiting software to keep the volume of music within safe levels. If your MP3 player doesn't come with this software already, it can sometimes be downloaded after purchase.'

Need2Know

## New European directive

In October 2009, the European Commission launched new hearing safety regulations regarding volume levels on MP3 players. All such players sold in the EU must have a default setting limiting the volume to 80 decibels. Exposure at this level is recommended to be no more than 40 hours a week.

While it is still possible to override this setting, manufacturers will have to provide clear warnings of the long-term adverse effects loud music can have on hearing.

The move follows research from 2008 which highlighted the need for personal music player manufacturers to control prolonged exposure to loud music. It was welcomed by organisations such as the British Tinnitus Association, which reports increasing numbers of people contacting them after developing tinnitus due to exposure to loud noise.

# Parenting a deaf child

No one is more expert in parenting your child than you are, and the decisions you make as a parent are so highly individual that it's hard to offer one-size-fits-all advice. So what follows should be regarded as a rough guide rather than a set of definitive answers.

# Hearing aids and children

Some children may get upset about having to wear hearing aids, or if other children ask about them. They may also become very distressed if the batteries run down, or if the hearing aid becomes lost or broken.

- While you can deal with the battery problem by always ensuring you or your child have some spares with you, especially for school, spare NHS hearing aids are rarely issued. If there is a problem with your child's aid, you will just have to reassure them and get the problem dealt with as soon as possible.

- In terms of explaining what hearing aids are to other children, clear, simple explanation will work best. Explain that your child's ears don't work very well, so they cannot hear properly and have to wear aids to help them, just as some people have to wear glasses if they can't see very well.

'Between 50 and 100 million people use personal music players every day and an estimated 10 million people in the EU could be left with hearing damage later in life as a result of listening to music at loud volumes and for prolonged periods of time, according to an EU scientific committee.'
British Tinnitus Association.

To get your child accustomed to hearing sound through an aid, try using play to encourage attentive listening. For example, create a tape of different sounds – sirens, a dog barking, water running, etc, and devise a game with picture cards that match the sounds, the object being to pair the sound to the right picture.

# Dealing with emotions

As the parent of a deaf child, you are likely, at various times, to experience a range of different emotions, including frustration, pride, anger, sorrow and elation – all the emotions, in fact, which any parent feels at one time or another. After all, the things which are good for deaf children are likely to be those which are good for all children.

Your child has to be able to communicate their emotions to you, however young they are. Try to think about how you might remove anything which is stopping this communication from taking place. Of course, words are not the only way to convey feelings – stories, books, facial expressions and gestures can also all be used. Some families have used photographs with happy or sad faces.

However you do it, it is important to include emotional vocabulary as you develop your child's language so that they have the tools to express themselves emotionally. Acknowledge your child's feelings, and let them know that these emotions are perfectly normal.

## Frustration

Some deaf children experience high levels of frustration which may be related to a lack of information, or frustration at not being able to communicate or express emotions. Of course, all children are frustrated occasionally, especially once they become teenagers.

With some deaf children, frustration may have a specific source, such as not being allowed to play outside because they cannot hear the traffic. Communication, negotiation and discussion and working to prevent or prepare for potentially frustrating situations will all help. Some parents find an activity such as a quiet walk will distract and calm their child, or developing other systems for taking time out or rewarding good behaviour.

It's also important that grandparents and any other carer of your child adopt a consistent approach so that the same rules apply whoever is looking after your child.

## Developing communication skills

If you develop your child's language and communication skills successfully, it will help all other aspects of parenting fall into place.

Whether you use sign language, speech or a combination of the two, there are strategies you can use to help develop your child's command of language, and with trial and error you can find something which works for you.

This might include building up a word or sign vocabulary, involving the child in all family situations and decisions, or using books or pictures. You can seize on any particular interest your child may have – for example, cars, trains or animals – and build up words and skills that way. Some parents find it helpful to put labels on objects around the house, or to make clay models of the words their child is learning.

Remember you will need to face your child when talking to them. Don't allow frustration to enter your voice, however many times you have to repeat yourself.

## Boosting confidence

It's understandable that you may feel an urge to overprotect your child. All parents feel this sometimes. It's important to remember that they need to develop their confidence, just as a hearing child does, and a confident child is likely to be a happier child.

There are many ways of building a child's confidence, and you will have to work out what works best for you. Here are some potential ideas:

- Teach your child how to explain to others that they have a hearing problem.

- Encourage them to speak for themselves as much as possible and to do as much for themselves as they can.

- Prepare for and rehearse different situations.

- Provide them with reassurance, approval and praise.

- Help them to understand that they will not always get their own way just because they are deaf.

- Find sporting or other activities which they enjoy and can become good at.

- Develop confidence in stages by doing small things first – like posting a letter or riding a bus alone. Some parents have found it helpful to give their child a note with their name, address and destination on it so they have a safety net if necessary.

You may also need to work on the confidence of grandparents or other family members in looking after your child. You may want to think about building up the amount of time someone else has exclusive care of your child, first for a few hours then overnight, for example. If grandparents or other carers have a basic understanding of how hearing aids work and how to change batteries, this can help improve their confidence levels as well.

# Mixing with others

Some parents may feel concerned that their deaf child could find it hard to mix with other children and that this could make them isolated. It is important that your son or daughter has contact with both deaf and hearing children.

Here are a few ideas which may help:

- Encourage friends to come to your house and allow your child to visit their friends' homes from an early age. If a hearing child spends time at your home, they will gain a greater understanding of what it means for your child to be deaf on a daily basis.

- Encourage others to talk to your child so they get used to people other than you.

- Encourage sports and other extra-curricular activities.

- Urge your child to socialise with just one other child or in small groups to start off with.

- Encourage friendships both at school and in your local community, especially if your child travels to a school some distance from your home, or if the children who live nearest to you attend different schools.

- Do journeys with your child before they have to make them themselves, letting them 'take' you, until they are familiar with the route and aware of any problems.

# Warning deaf children about danger

If you have a deaf child, warning them about danger can pose particular challenges. You will need good communication skills to explain that heat, sharp objects, stairs and roads can all be dangerous.

Signs on hot and cold household appliances, role play and play acting can all help.

# Dealing with a hearing sibling

If your deaf child has a brother or sister with good hearing, it's important that they don't feel left out, either in terms of the attention they deserve in their own right, or in terms of keeping them in the picture about their sibling's hearing loss.

Consultations with siblings through surveys and focus groups have shown that most brothers and sisters of deaf children wanted to know what was going on at hospital appointments, as well as information about what it means to be deaf and its implications for family life (NDCS, 2008). Some older siblings have reported that they would have liked more information earlier on, as this would have reduced the level of confusion and feelings of resentment, anger and, for some, isolation that they felt.

Of course, what you tell your children, and when, differs hugely from family to family, and it is very much an individual decision. Here are some hints and some frequently asked questions to help guide you.

'Encourage friendships both at school and in your local community, especially if your child travels to a school some distance from your home, or if the children who live nearest to you attend different schools.'

Q. Is there a particular age when they are most likely to be able to start understanding?

A. Every sibling will have a different story about when they first learnt they had a deaf brother or sister and understood what was going on. Recent work with siblings focus groups has found that hearing siblings under the age of seven may not have a good understanding of what is happening, and may not be able to express how they feel about having a deaf brother or sister (NDCS, 2008).

'When explaining to young siblings what deafness is and how the ear works, you could consider making a basic model of an ear out of toilet roll and yoghurt pots and talking about it.'

Q. How should you encourage a hearing sibling to behave towards a deaf child?

A. This depends on individual circumstances. It is important that the hearing sibling behaves in a positive way but does not shy away from their emotions and how they feel. Positive wellbeing of both the sibling and deaf child is very important, and having an unhappy sibling will affect the deaf child's life too.

Q. Is there anything you can do to stop hearing siblings feeling left out and does this happen often?

A. Talk to the sibling and explain what is happening. Research shows that those who have been involved in decisions about their deaf brother or sister, or were aware of the reasons for hospital visits, did not feel as left out as those who were unaware of what was happening.

Good, clear communication is key to ensuring the hearing sibling doesn't feel left out. It is important to spend a balance of time with both children.

Q. What can a hearing sibling do to help?

A. There are lots of things that a hearing sibling can do to help. Some siblings do this by supporting their parents, while others will make sure they communicate clearly and properly understand what deafness means and some of the frustrations of their deaf brother or sister.

**Case study**

Full-time mum Sam, 26, and husband John, 30, live with their non-identical twin sons Harvey and Ronnie in Clacton-on-Sea, Essex. Born in April 2008, both boys have the same level of hearing loss.

Sam says: 'Harvey and Ronnie were born nine weeks early. We first realised there was a problem with their hearing after their newborn hearing screen, when they were just a couple of weeks old in the special care baby unit. The test came back "non-responsive", but the nurse told us not to worry – easy for her to say!

'Finally, at around eight months old, a mild hearing loss in both boys was diagnosed at Colchester hospital. We were told they'd need hearing aids and were sent away in total shock at the thought of our beautiful boys having a hearing loss. John and I didn't speak about it at first. I think we thought that if we did we'd just get upset or angry.

'At 11 months, we were told that, although they had slight glue ear, there was a permanent hearing loss which had become moderate rather than mild, and hearing aids would be needed all their lives. It was very stressful, and inevitably I blamed myself. We were so shocked and sad for our boys.

'We found the website of the NDCS very helpful and went on one of their weekends for children newly diagnosed with hearing problems. It was lovely meeting other families and their children, and this was the first time we felt able to talk openly about the problem. Our own families have also been very supportive.

'We still don't know what the options are for the twins' education. A deaf teacher visits every month to play with them to see how they are getting on. We hope they will be able to attend a mainstream school.

'I don't think you ever deal emotionally with the fact that your children are hearing impaired, so I still have good and bad days. I'd still love them to be able to hear a simple sound like bath water running, but they are happy and healthy, so to me Ronnie and Harvey are perfect. I am so happy to be their mum, and so proud they are my children.'

# Summing Up

- Compared to adults, deaf children require a different approach and strategies from professionals to deal with their hearing loss.

- Childhood deafness covers the full spectrum of sound frequencies.

- Deafness in childhood can affect language, speech, social and educational development.

- There are various causes of childhood deafness, some of them temporary, for example glue ear, and others permanent.

- It's crucial for all newborn babies to have their hearing thoroughly tested.

- Ear protection is vital at concerts, in clubs and when listening to recorded music.

- There are plenty of ways to ensure you don't neglect the need of a hearing sibling if you have a deaf child.

- Think carefully about how best you can develop your child's language skills and their ability to communicate.

- Think about ways of discussing danger so that your child understands.

- Make sure they have a vocabulary for emotions and are able to express their feelings.

- Do everything possible to boost your child's confidence and to encourage independence and social interaction with deaf and hearing children.

# Chapter Three

## Glue Ear

Glue ear, or otitis media, is the single most common cause of deafness in younger children and can persist well into adolescence. In fact, it is one of the most frequently occurring childhood illnesses. It is estimated that up to a fifth of children aged between two and five are experiencing it at any one time.

Essentially, glue ear is a build-up of fluid in the middle ear which can become thick and sticky, hence the condition's name. However, not all children have this discharge, so, as a parent, you need to be alert to other symptoms as well. It can come and go in recurring bouts, making it much harder for a child to hear and process information.

Although glue ear is not in itself an infection, the fluid is a good breeding ground for infection, which can co-exist in some children. If the glue becomes infected, a burst eardrum may result and the pus may escape out of the ear via the ear canal.

For many children, glue ear is something which clears up quickly. But potentially, and especially if it persists, it can be a disruptive condition since it can affect a child's social and behavioural development, as well as their education. Research suggests that 1 in 20 five-year-olds could have long-lasting problems as a result of glue ear.

Left untreated, glue ear can have an impact on the speed with which a child develops literacy and language skills and their sense of balance. There is also research suggesting there could be a link between glue ear and dyslexia.

If undetected, children's behaviour can change so that they become withdrawn and appear to lose concentration. Sometimes, this can be mistaken for stubbornness or rudeness.

Glue ear can occur in one or both of a child's ears; if it is experienced in both ears, it is described as bilateral otitis media.

Good hearing requires the ear's airways to be clear, and glue ear occurs when the sticky glue-like fluid produced by cells lining the middle ear builds up. This blocks the Eustachian tube, which tends to be narrower in young children, so that hearing becomes very limited.

## Causes of glue ear

No one really knows why some children get this condition, although some causes of glue ear have been suggested. These include passive smoking, allergies (e.g. to milk) and the idea that glue ear may run in families. Links have also been made with cold weather and the bacteria which come with colds, flu or sore throats. Equally, children with a cleft lip or palate, or Down's syndrome, are thought to be disproportionately more likely to have glue ear.

'There are proven links with glue ear and ear infections and heavy colds. Often, glue ear can clear up once a bad cold has gone.'

Additionally, there are proven links with glue ear and ear infections and heavy colds. Often, glue ear can clear up once a bad cold has gone.

There is some evidence to suggest that breastfeeding could lessen the chances of glue ear developing. Breast milk has proteins which are thought to help stop inflammation and protect against glue ear even after an infant is no longer breastfed.

## Types of glue ear

Essentially, glue ear takes one of three basic forms.

### Common glue ear, or otitis media with effusion

This is the least severe type. There are various symptoms, including:

- Tiredness.

- Appearing not to hear.

- Earache, sometimes with discharge.

- Withdrawn, clinging or persistently protesting behaviour – frustration and social difficulties.

- Lack of concentration.
- Restlessness at night.
- Breathing through the mouth rather than the nose.
- Frequent colds.

## Chronic otitis media

A child who has chronic glue ear is likely to have some or all of the above symptoms, sometimes with a thick and smelly discharge from their ear and longer-term hearing problems.

## Acute otitis media

This is the condition in its severest form. A child experiencing it could have severe earache, a high temperature, a tendency to tug repeatedly on their ears and a general feeling of being unwell. The eardrum may burst which will relieve the pain and there may be discharge of blood-stained pus from the ear.

If, along with the symptoms described above, there also seem to be problems with your child's learning process, including things like poor concentration, a weak vocabulary or difficulties with reading and basic maths, you should talk to the special educational needs co-ordinator (SENCO) at your child's school as soon as possible. The school, or your GP or health visitor, may also be able to refer you to a speech and language therapist.

# Treatment of glue ear

Most children will grow out of glue ear eventually, but while a child has the problem, it can affect their development. A specialist ear, nose and throat (ENT) doctor will monitor chronic and acute glue ear to prevent complications, including permanent deafness.

'Most children will grow out of glue ear eventually, but while a child has the problem, it can affect their development. A specialist ear, nose and throat (ENT) doctor will monitor chronic and acute glue ear to prevent complications, including permanent deafness.'

There are many things which can be done to treat glue ear and opinions on how best to do this have changed over the years. Some doctors prefer to allow the condition to clear up untreated. Antibiotics will not clear up glue ear but may be prescribed if there's an ear infection at the same time. Sometimes decongestants, nasal sprays, ear drops or pain-killers are also used.

Another idea is the use of an 'otovent' – a small plastic device with a little balloon which a child blows up through its nose, with the aim of opening the Eustachian tube.

Equally, some doctors may prefer to refer a child for a hearing test, also known as a tympanometry test. This assesses a child's hearing by measuring the extent to which the middle ear can move. The graph the test produces offers an immediate result.

While older children may well be referred for a full hearing test, 'distraction' tests are an option for younger children under four, although the accuracy of these kinds of tests is variable.

Bear in mind that glue ear and the hearing difficulties it brings fluctuate a lot – a child who hears perfectly well one week may not do so the next. So an accurate diagnosis of glue ear cannot be made on the basis of one hospital visit.

## Treatment with surgery

If alternative treatments don't help clear up glue ear, surgery may well be suggested as an option. Of course, no surgery is entirely risk free, and the decision to operate on a child is not one to be taken lightly.

Surgery for glue ear offers temporary relief from the condition, so if the condition returns or is severe it may be necessary to repeat the procedure. Repeated surgery for glue ear can sometimes cause the eardrum to scar, causing mild but permanent hearing loss. So doctors may advise leaving surgery until children are slightly older, especially if there is a risk of recurring glue ear.

Generally speaking, surgery for glue ear, involving the insertion of small tubes or grommets, is a straightforward procedure carrying very little risk. During the surgery, the doctor will drain the fluid from the ear, and the grommets then allow free flow of air inside the ear and stop more fluid building up.

'Generally speaking, surgery for glue ear, involving the insertion of small tubes or grommets, is a straightforward procedure carrying very little risk.'

Quite often, it is possible for children to have their adenoids removed at the same time as this procedure is carried out. Typically, this is done while the second or third set of grommets is fitted, rather than the first.

Results from this procedure tend to be almost instantaneous and on average grommets can stay in place for six to nine months. They usually fall out on their own and cause no further problems. Very occasionally, your ENT doctor may have to remove them, but this is rare.

In some cases, while children are waiting to see if glue ear corrects itself naturally, or while waiting for the grommets operation, their hearing can be affected for an extended period. To ensure there is no negative impact on speech and education during this time, you may want to think about hearing aids or ask for additional support at school – which may be something as simple as making sure your child sits as close to the teacher as possible.

# While your child has grommets in place

- Try not to let your child place their head underwater, at least without a swimming hat.

- When hair washing, Vaseline on cotton wool will stop water from getting into the ear.

- If your child has a milk allergy which seems to be making their glue ear worse, stick to a dairy-free alternative until the condition has cleared. (But do seek medical and nutritional advice before doing this.)

# Complementary remedies

Some complementary treatments are supported by slim or very poor evidence. Sometimes this may simply be because they are new, although alternative and complementary treatments do not tend to have the backing of sound scientific research evidence.

In February 2008, NICE published a clinical guideline about the surgical management of otitis media with effusion in children. It makes recommendations about:

- The complete assessment of children, including the tests which should be carried out to diagnose the condition.

- Which children will benefit from surgical intervention.

- The effectiveness of surgical and non-surgical interventions.

- The management of otitis media with effusion in children with Down's syndrome and those with a cleft palate.

The non-surgical treatments which NICE considered included:

- The use of antibiotics.

- Antihistamines.

- Decongestants.

- Steroids.

- Immunostimulants.

- The use of therapies such as cranial osteopathy, homeopathy, acupuncture and massage.

NICE found no evidence to support the use of any of these interventions, and no evidence that changes to diet will improve this condition. It recommends that hearing aids should be offered to children with persistent bilateral otitis media effusion and hearing loss as an alternative to surgical intervention where surgery is not an appropriate option.

You can read the guideline in full by visiting http://guidance.nice.org.uk/CG60. If you think your child is eligible for treatment but it's not been made available, see www.nice.org.uk/aboutguidance.

## How you can help your child with glue ear

- Reinforce the work of your child's school. Communicate well with teachers and share information.

- Make sure you have your child's attention before talking to them, and are always facing them. You don't need to make exaggerated mouth movements – just speak clearly. Minimise background noise when speaking and crouch down to the child's level to talk.

- Show older children how non-verbal signals such as body language, eye contact and facial expression can help with communication.

# Speech and language development

Part of the way we learn speech is biological, but we also learn to speak by interacting with others. Children are most likely to acquire language well during the first four years of life and will go through various stages of language development.

For many children, glue ear strikes at the very age when they most need to be able to hear well to acquire language skills. For example, they may miss out parts of words when speaking. Consequently, the condition means they may not develop these abilities with the same speed as their peers do.

Differing levels of hearing loss will affect a child's learning and behaviour as well as the way they respond to and interact with their environment. Glue ear can cause tiredness, pain, withdrawal and lethargy, and can also make a child easily distracted and clingy. It's all too easy for a child with this condition to fall behind in their early development.

Teachers and parents should join forces with a speech and language therapist if necessary to highlight weaknesses and put together a programme of intervention with the aim of stopping the child from falling behind at school.

Both home and classroom environments should allow children to function properly despite the difficulties.

'Differing levels of hearing loss will affect a child's learning and behaviour as well as the way they respond to and interact with their environment. Glue ear can cause tiredness, pain, withdrawal and lethargy, and can also make a child easily distracted and clingy.'

# Summing Up

- Glue ear is the commonest cause of childhood deafness and is a build-up of fluid in the middle ear which can occur in one or both ears. There are three basic forms and it is usually a temporary problem.

- No one really understands why some children get glue ear, although several theories have been put forward.

- If it is not treated, glue ear can affect a child's behaviour and language and literacy development as well as their hearing.

- There are many things which can be done to treat glue ear and to help the children who have it.

- Surgery is a safe option and involves the insertion of grommets or small tubes which drain the built-up fluid.

- Close co-operation and communication with your child's school will be invaluable in their development.

- Glue ear should be monitored by a doctor at all times.

# Chapter Four
## Education

### What are special educational needs?

A child is considered to have special educational needs if they have a learning difficulty or disability which makes it harder for them to learn than most other children at the same stage of their academic career.

Special educational needs could mean behavioural, medical, learning, emotional or communication problems, as well as a sensory issue such as a hearing loss or visual impairment. Children have varying types and levels of special educational needs and learn at different paces and in their own ways.

If your child has not yet started school or pre-school, your first port of call should be your doctor or health visitor, with whom you can discuss any concerns. They can offer advice on the next steps to take and who to go to for help.

If your child is already at school, nursery or pre-school, talk first to their class teacher and/or the school's SENCO. The SENCO's job is to oversee help for all children who have special educational needs. They will be able to tell you what the school thinks and what will happen next. They can give you information and help to put your mind at rest.

It is in the best interests of both children and parents to work in co-operation with teachers. The more closely you liaise with your child's teachers, the more effective any help is likely to be. The school should keep you fully informed about your child's progress every step of the way.

Equally, for further information you are entitled to see the school's policy on special educational needs and the school's annual report.

'I like Travel and Tourism best, and would like to do a two-year catering course at college then work for P&O Ferries.'

Jo, Henry Beaufort School, Winchester.

# Early educational setting

The emphasis is on early identification and help with a graduated approach; in other words, gently increasing the amount of help given.

Extra help your child receives because of their hearing loss is called Early Years Action or School Action, and parents must be informed that this action is being given.

If your child is still not progressing as they should, the SENCO should discuss with you the possibility of calling in external help, such as a specialist teacher. This type of help is known as Early Years Action Plus or School Action Plus. Your child's progress will be carefully recorded, monitored and reviewed. As your child has a hearing difficulty, you should always ask that your child is monitored by a qualified teacher of the deaf.

It is part of the SENCO's role to involve you as much as possible and take your views into account when making any decisions, while also letting you know about your child's progress every step of the way.

There should be a clear written record about what the early years setting or school has done to assess and provide for your child's needs, which should be discussed with you. There will be an education plan for your child and reference to the involvement of other professionals, where relevant.

'It is part of the SENCO's role to involve you as much as possible and take your views into account when making any decisions, while also letting you know about your child's progress every step of the way.'

# The assessment process

If your son or daughter does not appear to be making the right progress at school, and the school, pre-school or nursery cannot provide everything your child needs, the local authority (LA) may carry out a statutory assessment of your child's needs.

Every LA has a different way of funding its schools. In some areas, schools are expected to fund all the extra help your child needs. In others, schools may only be expected to fund some of the extra support. LAs also have different policies about how schools are able to access specialist support, for example specialist teachers and/or speech and language therapists. It is therefore impossible to say when you should think that such an assessment is the way forward for your child. LAs have to explain this SEN information on their website.

Generally speaking, only around 2% of the whole school population needs a statutory assessment, so it will only be needed for children with the severest and most long-term hearing difficulties.

When the LA is asked to carry out an assessment, either by a parent or school, it has six weeks in which to make a decision on whether to do so, although there are some specific exceptions to this rule.

The LA should write to you and:

- Tell you it is deciding whether to do a statutory assessment.

- Explain what happens next and how long the assessment will take.

- Give you a named officer at the LA as your point of contact.

- Tell you about the Parent Partnership Service who can offer independent advice and support.

- Ask both you and the school for your views about your child's special educational needs and details of anyone you would like the LA to talk to about your child.

If an assessment is necessary, they will ask various professionals to give their thoughts on your child, including:

- Your child's early education setting or school.

- An educational psychologist.

- A doctor.

- A hearing professional.

- Social services or therapists (if necessary).

Your views will be sought again. You will also need to think about which school you want your child to attend. You can also recommend any other people or organisations whose views could help in the assessment of your child. The LA will also ask what your child thinks themselves about their special educational needs.

'I've always been deaf so it's not really a difficulty. I'd like to be a chef, a mechanic or a train driver. I like technology and the lessons, staff and students at the deaf unit best. It's good being able to turn off my hearing aid when it's noisy!'

Alex, Henry Beaufort School, Winchester.

There shouldn't be more than 10 weeks between the date the assessment is first requested and the issue of any final statement.

Once the LA has all the information it needs, it can decide whether to make a Statement of Special Educational Needs for your child.

This legal document is a detailed guide to:

- Your child's special educational needs.

- The educational provision which will meet those needs.

- Any other arrangements which will help your child.

Anyone reading the statement should be able to understand from it everything that may be linked to your child's hearing loss.

Statements are set out in six parts:

- Section 1 gives information about your child.

- Section 2 describes the difficulties your child has, and their needs.

- Section 3 outlines the special help your child will receive, including for speech and language difficulties.

- Section 4 names the school and the kind of educational provision your child will receive.

- Section 5 discusses any non-educational needs your child may have.

- Section 6 describes the help which will meet those needs.

You will be able to see and comment on a draft statement before the document is finalised. You can also meet the LA to discuss it if you wish.

You can disagree with all or some of the statement, and must make your comments on the draft statement within two weeks, then any further points must be made at no later than two weeks after that.

Within eight weeks of issuing the draft, the LA must finalise the statement. It comes into effect immediately.

# Statement of Special Educational Needs annual review

Every year, the LA has to review your child's Statement of Special Educational Needs.

This review:

- Collates the views of everyone helping your child.
- Assesses how successful the statement has been to date.
- Looks ahead with fresh targets for the coming year.

## What if I am still worried?

If you are still concerned that your child's needs are not being met, there are things you can do.

In the first instance, you should talk to either the SENCO at your child's school or your child's class teacher. Remember, even if things can seem frustrating at times, and appear to move too slowly, it is important for you to co-operate with your child's school.

Many LAs also have other sources of support, such as the Parent Partnership Service, or you may find local voluntary or parents' groups which are also supportive.

## Appealing against a special educational needs decision

If you do not agree with the decision which your LA has made about your child's education, you have the right to appeal against it. However, this should probably be considered a last resort, after you have tried other approaches.

If you do decide to appeal, you have two months after receiving the final written decision from your LA in which to do so. And, even then it's still worth attempting to resolve things with your LA yourself.

Appeals are considered by SENDIST – the Special Educational Needs and Disability Discrimination Tribunal, which provides a free service. You can find more about this organisation at www.sendist.gov.uk.

The tribunal is an independent body, with no connection to government or any LA. Three appointed members consider individual appeals. The panel is chaired by a tribunal judge, who will be a lawyer, and the two other members are non-legal specialists who understand special educational needs and disability. Sometimes, the judge is able to make a decision alone, but this process, or 'hearing', is still known as a tribunal.

'Making an appeal can seem a daunting process. You may be able to get help from a parents' group or other voluntary group as you make your appeal.'

## When should I appeal?

You may wish to consider an appeal if:

- You have asked for the LA to carry out a statutory assessment but they have not done this.

- The LA refuses to make a Statement of Special Educational Needs following an assessment.

- There has been no re-assessment of your child's needs for six months or more.

- Your child's statement is cancelled.

- You disagree with how your child's needs are described, the educational provision which has been recommended or the school or type of school named in the statement.

- The LA has not named a school in the statement.

## How do I appeal?

You can find the appeal form on the SENDIST website – you have to complete and return it. Your appeal will then be registered and acknowledged within 10 working days. The LA will receive a copy of your appeal and then has 30 working days to respond – you should get a copy of their response.

Making an appeal can seem a daunting process. You may be able to get help from a parents' or other voluntary group as you make your appeal.

At least 10 working days before it takes place, SENDIST will inform you of the venue and time of your hearing. One or both parents can attend, as well as the child if they want to, along with up to three witnesses.

You can claim reasonable travel expenses for you and your witnesses to attend the hearing, and witnesses may be able to claim a fixed amount for loss of earnings.

If you are a deaf or hearing impaired parent and need a British Sign Language (BSL) interpreter or lipspeaker, the tribunal will provide this.

You should receive the tribunal's decision no later than 10 working days after the hearing.

An LA must implement the decision within a fixed period of the date the decision is made. If the LA doesn't comply, you may have to make a further appeal to the High Court, or complain to the Secretary of State for Children, Schools and Families.

## Further appeals

If you disagree with the tribunal's decision because you feel it is wrong in law, or for some other reason, you can appeal to the Administrative Appeals Chamber of the Upper Tribunal, but you need permission to do this first.

You should receive a leaflet explaining how to do this. Your options will also be outlined in detail when you receive the tribunal's decision.

# SEN Code of Practice

The government issued the SEN Code of Practice in 2001 which both SENDIST and every LA 'must have regard to'. You can read this document from the Department for Children, Schools and Families (DCSF), their address is at the back of the book. Alternatively, visit www.teachernet.gov.

# Educational options for deaf children

All LAs are obliged to provide for all children within their area, including those who are deaf or who have a hearing impairment, at primary and secondary level. Most will offer deaf provision within reasonable reach of everyone in its area.

One of the biggest decisions to be made is whether your child should be supported within a mainstream school, as part of a deaf unit in a mainstream school or taught in a specialist school for the deaf.

Equally, another big decision is how your child will communicate in class. The importance of strong communication is stressed in Every Child Matters, the government's initiative on the wellbeing of children and young people up to the age of 19.

The debate about whether to use sign language exclusively, oral forms of communication or a combination of both has been a heated one. The tendency in recent times has been towards 'total communication', involving a mix of sign language and other means of communicating.

Where speech and lipreading are involved, the method of teaching is known as oralism. Within the Deaf community – spelt deliberately with a capital D and referring to those who view deafness as a difference to be celebrated rather than a disability to be 'cured' – this form of education is sometimes frowned upon. Members of the Deaf community view sign language as a pivotal part of their identity and dislike what they see as attempts in schools to suppress its use.

And, of course, modern technology offers more ways of supporting the deaf child in the classroom than ever before.

The needs of deaf pupils may change over time and they may need to have access to various different communication modes.

Clearly each child's needs are different, with a different type and level of hearing loss, so support should be tailored to the individual pupil.

Need2Know

# Aids to communicating in school

A deaf child in school could use one or more of the following aids to communication:

- A note-taker, teaching assistant or sign language interpreter sitting with them in school.
- Radio aids which work in conjunction with hearing aids to pick up sound.
- A PA system, which may be especially useful in a situation such as a school assembly.
- Laptops such as Toughbooks from Panasonic, which are designed to withstand robust handling, can pick up what is being said from a distance and allow independent working in class.
- Sound field voice reinforcement systems use speakers and a surround system in the classroom to carry the teacher's voice and amplify it with minimum distortion.
- Learning and communication support assistants (CSAs) can also offer support, and are trained to at least Level 2 in British Sign Language.
- For a child with a hearing loss, it is crucial that, wherever they are being taught, the school communicates well with parents about how a child is doing and keeps detailed reports of progress.
- In many deaf units, pupils can spend time with a teacher before or after school to be sure they are fully prepared for lessons and have understood what they need to do for homework and so on.

### Case study

Henry Beaufort School in Winchester, Hampshire, is a comprehensive school specialising in teaching technology and has just under 1,000 pupils. Seven profound or severely deaf youngsters attend its hearing impaired unit. Henry Beaufort's latest OFSTED inspection described the school's pastoral care as 'outstanding' and its support for hearing impaired students as 'a strength'.

Pupils take part in a wide range of after-school activities and sporting and social events run by local and national deaf organisations – from scuba diving to cooking. Hearing impaired students also run deaf awareness training for Year 7 pupils.

Ruth Edwards heads the unit, where staff have been trained to work both orally and with children who use sign language. She says: 'Deaf children frequently have to work harder than their hearing counterparts just to make sure they take everything in, and so are likely to be very tired after school, especially if they have come in early or stayed on after class.

'Our deaf students don't get special treatment, but they do get all the support they need to reach their potential and to help their confidence and self-esteem grow.

'We offer a range of communication options and tailor support to individual needs. There are support assistants working in the classroom, who support our deaf students in a variety of ways, for example in using a remote tough book to assist independent learning.

'We encourage our students to aim high and we're very aware that our young people get only one chance to have an education. Our former pupils include an artist in residence, a musician and an IT technician. We tell everyone that having a hearing loss needn't stand in the way of success.

'With the advancement of technology such as digital hearing aids, support from national deaf organisations and government legislation including Every Child Matters, deaf students are much more included and able to achieve their personal best and reach their potential in life.'

> **Case study**
>
> 14-year-old female pupil at Henry Beaufort School
>
> 'I'm doing 12 subjects for my GCSEs and like art and English best. My ambition when I leave is to study to be a vet – I love looking after my pets at home.
>
> 'The best thing about school is meeting other deaf young people. At primary school, they used to call me names like "deafie" or "deaffo". When I was younger, my hearing kept getting worse and worse but for the last six years or so it has stayed more or less the same.
>
> 'It does annoy me, having a hearing problem. I wear two hearing aids and can hear the teacher most of the time. Sometimes, I have someone sitting next to me in the lesson. My friends help me if I get stuck.'

# Higher education

The next section deals with higher education and is aimed directly at students. However, if you're reading this as a parent please read on – there is plenty of important information relevant to parenting teenagers with a hearing impairment.

## Disabled Students' Allowance

This government grant covers extra expenses faced by disabled students as a direct result of being on a course of higher education.

As a student with a hearing impairment, you will be entitled to a Disabled Students' Allowance (DSA) if you are registered full time on an undergraduate degree programme, or a part-time student registered on at least 50% of an undergraduate degree programme. Awards for post-graduates are discretionary.

The DSA is made up of:

- The basic allowance – this is a yearly sum to cover extra living costs or small items of equipment.

- Large equipment allowance – these could be computers, radio aids or similar items. The maximum amount is currently £5,161 for your whole course.

- Non-Medical Personal Assistance Allowance – this is for personal help related to your programme of study. For a deaf or hearing impaired student, it could be used to pay for note-takers or sign language interpreters.

## Applying for DSA

Apply as soon as you can, wherever and whatever you are going to study.

The application form you need to complete, DSA1, may well be available from your university. If not, simply download a copy from the Direct Gov website. Along with the form, you will need to submit medical proof of disability – this could be a GP's letter, for example.

Your LA will consider the application and ask you to have a DSA needs assessment carried out at an assessment centre. Your needs and the results of your DSA assessment should guide your college or university.

If you live in Northern Ireland, Scotland or Wales and are studying anywhere in the UK, your application for student finance will be dealt with in your own region.

## How can your college or university help?

Your institution could provide:

- A hearing loop system in key teaching areas.
- Portable loops.
- Permission for you to have assistance dogs with you on campus.
- Vibrating pillows and flashing alarms in campus accommodation.
- Special doorbells in university-managed accommodation.

- Note-takers.

- British Sign Language interpreters.

- Lipspeakers.

- Horseshoe seating arrangements in learning settings.

- Social and/or academic mentor.

- Transcribed or sub-titled course materials.

- Tutor awareness of the situation and a willingness to understand, repeat information which has been missed and to spend more time with the deaf student to be sure everything has been taken in.

- Some institutions will also provide students eligible for DSA with an individual learning agreement, setting out their specific needs in a single document while also providing guidance to academic staff.

## The Quality Assurance Agency for Higher Education

The Quality Assurance Agency for Higher Education safeguards quality and standards across higher education in the UK. It has a code of practice about how universities should cater for students with any kind of disability, including hearing loss.

The measurement of quality of an institution's overall provision takes into account how well it meets the expectations of this code. This covers a wide range of issues surrounding university life – from equality of the application process to exams and the accessibility of support services.

A full copy is available from the Quality Assurance Agency for Higher Education's website (see help list).

At the same time, the Disability Discrimination Act (DDA) stresses that universities must publish a clear statement of their policy on ensuring equality for students with disabilities, so ask to see a copy of your university's policy.

## Life on campus

Without the right support, the university or college campus can be a potentially intimidating and isolating environment, especially for a student who is profoundly or severely deaf.

Particular support may be needed when someone first leaves home to start campus life, especially for students from a non-hearing background or family. Coping mechanisms which worked perfectly well before may not be so helpful in a university setting.

With a relatively short academic year, students often pack a lot into each term. But as a deaf student, you may find life even more tiring than your hearing colleagues, so you need to take particular care to pace yourself.

However, student life can be frustrating and exhausting at times whether or not you have a disability, and not all the problems deaf students come across are exclusive to them. Most students are coping with a new environment and being away from home for the first time, whether they can hear or not.

'With the right preparation and support, there is no reason you should not get as much out of your university career as anyone else.'

With the right preparation and support, there is no reason why you should not get as much out of your university career as anyone else.

Dr Lesley Black, head of disabilities and learning diversity at the University of Winchester, says: 'If you're thinking about college or university, research the subject and institution you are interested in as thoroughly as possible.

'Visit the campus, meet faculty members and the disability team, talk to students already there if you can. All these things will help a prospective student to get a feel for the particular place, and hopefully they will then feel more confident about putting in an application.

'I would always urge a full disclosure of the disability and any areas where support will be needed. I'd also encourage prospective students to apply for DSA well before arriving on campus so that support is already in place from day one.'

50

# Did you know?

Whether you have a hearing loss or not, if you became really interested in the subject, you could consider taking Deaf Studies at university, either at undergraduate or post-graduate level. The University of Reading offers a BA in Theatre Arts, Education and Deaf Studies, Bristol has a Centre for Deaf Studies, the University of Central Lancashire has offered a programme of Deaf Studies since 1993, while at City University London, the MSc in Human Communication includes specialist modules in Deaf Studies.

---

**Case study**

Nicola, 18, is studying for A-levels in graphics, art and photography at the specialist Mary Hare School near Newbury, Berkshire. She lost her hearing and became profoundly deaf aged 14 months.

'We are helped to hear at school by headphones in lessons and mostly we use a smart board. I have a mixture of deaf and hearing friends.

'I communicate with both sign language and speaking, but I don't use sign language with my family. I have used sign language since I was four. Using it makes me feel relaxed, and it is the best thing about being deaf! It makes it easy to communicate with deaf people socially. Although it's a struggle sometimes, I'm happy for who I am.'

---

# Summing Up

- Your child may be assessed for a Statement of Special Educational Needs.

- If you are in disagreement with your LA and what they have decided about your child's education, you can appeal against their decision.

- It's crucial to communicate well with your child's school at all stages.

- The school and LA must keep you fully informed at all stages of any assessment and appeal process and about any decisions made about your child's education.

- There are many options for your child's education and for how they will communicate with teachers and other pupils while they are in school.

- As a deaf student in higher education, it's important to claim for the DSA as soon as you can.

- There may well be challenges, but there are many things which your college or university can do to make life easier while you are with them.

# Chapter Five

# Deafness and Hearing Loss at Work

Under the DDA, it is against the law for employers to discriminate against anyone with any kind of disability, including a sensory impairment such as a hearing loss.

The DDA, as amended in 2005, clearly states that a disabled person is someone with 'a physical or mental impairment which has a substantial, long-term adverse effect on their ability to carry out normal day-to-day activities.'

For the purposes of the DDA:

- Substantial means neither minor nor trivial.

- Long-term means that the effect of the impairment has lasted or is likely to last for at least a year (special rules apply to recurring or fluctuating conditions).

- A normal day-to-day activity must affect one of the 'capacities' listed in the DDA, which includes hearing.

The DDA doesn't cover just the time you are working with your employer, but also the entire recruitment process, and things like:

- Promotion, transfer or training opportunities.

- Access to workplace benefits including recreational or refreshment facilities.

It is also unlawful to discriminate on grounds of disability during a redundancy or dismissal process.

'Under the DDA, it is against the law for employers to discriminate against anyone with any kind of disability, including a sensory impairment such as a hearing loss.'

The DDA means that your employer has an absolute, non-negotiable duty to provide 'reasonable adjustments' so that your working arrangements do not put you at a disadvantage because of your disability.

The key word here is 'reasonable', which is open to fairly broad interpretation. If an employer deems that an adjustment would be unreasonable, then they are not under any obligation to make it. There is no definitive list, but in general terms 'reasonable adjustments' cover a broad range of things, and could feasibly include:

- Allowing an employee extra time to complete a task.
- Adjustments to a workplace building.
- Providing a reader, interpreter or other support worker.
- Providing more accessible instructions.
- Allocating some of an employee's duties to a colleague.

The biggest concern, particularly for small businesses, has traditionally been the expense involved in making adjustments to a building or hiring support staff. But each case is unique, and the adjustments must be appropriate both to the job an employee is doing, as well as an individual's needs. For example, a specially adapted telephone would not necessarily be a reasonable adjustment for a cleaner whose job didn't involve long telephone conversations.

For someone who is deaf or hearing impaired, specific 'reasonable adjustments' could cover things like:

- A specially adapted telephone.
- A loop system for meeting rooms.
- Time off to attend lip reading or BSL classes.
- Provision of a BSL interpreter or lipspeaker where appropriate.
- Microphone equipment for meetings.
- Confirmation of instructions in writing, use of email and text messaging rather than speech where possible and avoiding use of mobile phones.
- Holding meetings in quieter rooms where possible.

'Remember, as well as being under an obligation to make "reasonable adjustments", employers must also not subject the employee to any kind of discrimination or treat them in any way differently from any other employee because of their disability.'

- Inclusion of subtitles for things like training or other work-related DVDs.

- Willingness to use a textphone where appropriate.

- Use of one-to-one communication rather than group meetings where possible.

- Provision of written copies of presentations or meetings which have been conducted orally.

- Willingness of managers to repeat themselves where necessary.

- Holding recruitment interviews in a well-lit room, allowing deaf candidates to sit next to the interview panel and making interviewers aware of the problem.

## Talking to your employer

While it is the legal obligation of the employer to make the right adjustments so that someone with a hearing difficulty can do their job properly, it is just as important for the employee to play their part in the working relationship. This means, for example, researching what equipment may be best for you at work and being prepared to try new things.

Equally, while this may sound very basic, it is also your responsibility to make sure you wear your hearing aid and have spare batteries with you at work. You should always feel able to ask a colleague or a manager to repeat things you have missed, especially instructions, rather than simply hoping for the best.

Understandably, disclosure of a hearing problem to an employer or a potential employer can seem a thorny issue; many people are reluctant to discuss their hearing loss at work. However, the sooner you declare your hearing difficulty, the sooner you can enjoy the legal protection to which you are entitled.

No employer can do anything to help any member of staff if they do not know about a problem. So it pays to be as honest and as open as you can from the outset, both about the extent and nature of your loss and how best you think your employer can help you.

Remember, the law covers you from the moment you start filling in your application form for a job, and an employer is not allowed to discriminate at any stage of the recruitment process or at any time while you are working for them.

'There are lots of things you can do if you feel you are being discriminated against, or that your employer isn't making the "reasonable adjustments" you need at your workplace, resulting in your performance being affected as a result. You don't have to suffer in silence.'

## What can I do if my employer won't listen?

The law may be in place but that doesn't stop discrimination at work from taking place against some deaf and hearing impaired employees.

Discrimination can take many direct and indirect forms: from a refusal to repeat something or making meetings inaccessible, to expressing exasperation and a lack of understanding that the deaf colleague can't hear on a mobile phone.

There are lots of things you can do if you feel you are being discriminated against, or that your employer isn't making the 'reasonable adjustments' you need at your workplace and this is affecting your performance. You don't have to suffer in silence.

The first thing you should do is chat to your immediate manager or colleague who you believe is behind the discrimination. Try to sort things out with them informally, but if you are struggling to get anywhere, talk to your human resources department or a senior colleague. Explain the situation as clearly and as honestly as you can, and try and come up with some sensible suggestions as to how things can be improved.

If you feel you are being bullied or discriminated against because of your hearing problem, it's important to keep a very detailed written record of specific examples of this.

If you are not already a member of a union, you might want to think about joining one. Other organisations able to help include the Citizens' Advice Bureau (CAB) and the Advisory, Conciliation and Arbitration Service (ACAS), which runs a confidential helpline. In severe cases, you may also wish to think about seeking the advice of an employment lawyer.

An employment tribunal is a way of taking your employer to court if you feel you've tried everything but discrimination has persisted and your employer has failed to comply with their legal obligations.

However, a tribunal should be viewed as a worst case scenario and as a last resort. The decision to go down this route is not one to be taken lightly and you have many options before things get to this stage.

If you really feel you have no alternative, the website of the Law Society is a good place to start looking for an employment lawyer and league tables of law firms are also available. Chamber and Partners has a guide, and you may also find it helpful to contact the Disability Law Service (see help list for details).

# Access to work in practice

When discussing adjustments at work with your employer, there are several things to take into consideration. You both need to think about how effective any adjustment will be, how practical it will be to bring about and how significantly it will reduce the problems your hearing loss causes.

Is it affordable? Will it cause much disruption to colleagues? Will it help any other people at work? How quickly and easily can the adjustment be installed?

Access to Work is a programme run by Jobcentre Plus offering advice on appropriate adjustments at work for anyone with a disability and often financial help as well. The programme supports all employers and employees and covers a wide range of different disabilities.

If you believe that your work is likely to be affected by a disability or health condition which will probably last a year or longer, get in touch with your regional Access to Work centre to see whether you may qualify for assistance.

The disability employment adviser (DEA) at your local Jobcentre will also be able to tell you about Access to Work.

## How it works

You'll need to return a straightforward application form, then an Access to Work adviser will normally speak to both you and your employer to decide which support would be best for you. While this can often be done over the phone, your adviser may visit you at work and have the discussion in person. Clearly, if you have a hearing loss, this may be the best option for you.

'If you believe that your work is likely to be affected by a disability or health condition likely to last a year or longer, get in touch with your regional Access to Work centre to see whether you may qualify for assistance.'

If your adviser feels specialist advice is appropriate, they may contact a specialist organisation to complete an assessment and recommend the right support.

Once your adviser has decided what support should be made available and Jobcentre Plus has approved this, they will write to you and your employer to tell you what has been decided and what support and grant you are entitled to.

The level of assistance Access to Work could give you will depend on how long you've been with your employer and whether you work for yourself.

You may receive all of the approved costs of the support if you are:

- Beginning a new job after a period of unemployment.
- Self-employed.
- Employed and have been in your job less than six weeks.

Access to Work will also pay up to 100% of the approved costs of help with:

- Support workers.
- Fares to work.
- Communicator support at interview.

If the following apply to you, Access to Work is only able to help with a proportion of the costs:

- You're already employed.
- You've been doing your job for six weeks or longer.
- Special equipment or adaptations to premises are needed.

Access to Work and your employer will agree exactly how the costs of providing you with the support you need are to be divided.

Access to Work will review your situation at work and the support you're getting between one and three years later.

## Case study

Mary's story

'I had been happily employed in the communications department of a large firm for nearly three years and found most people sympathetic to my hearing loss. I relied on email and face-to-face meetings wherever possible. I also had a specially adapted phone and used a microphone in meetings.

'Then my boss changed and so did my role; things took a turn for the worse. My boss was often impatient and repeatedly tried to speak to me by shouting from a mobile phone from a moving car with loud motorway sounds in the background. She tended to raise her voice thinking that would help me to hear better, when it actually had the opposite effect.

'She also told me that I "shouldn't be working in communications", and said "don't give me any of that politically correct nonsense" when I protested, and complained that I was "as useful as a chocolate teapot".

'I tolerated the situation for some months, unsure of what to do. Other colleagues noticed the bad behaviour. Eventually, I spoke to human resources and my Staff Association, who between them secured a compromise agreement. This meant that I agreed to leave my job in return for a sum of money, and would bring no further action.

'While my solicitor pointed out that I could have taken the case further, I decided I wanted to avoid the stress of a court case and to get on with my life. But it still makes me sad that it meant the end of a job I'd always previously enjoyed. It certainly didn't feel like much of a victory at the time.

'I would urge anyone who is experiencing problems at work to take action and seek advice as quickly as possible.'

## Case study

Mark: a landmark case

Mark, 40, a deaf man from Grantham who was refused a job because of his disability, won his fight to prove he was the victim of discrimination under the DDA in a landmark case.

The former Disability Rights Commission (the DRC, whose responsibilities have since transferred to the new Equality and Human Rights Commission) acted for Mark in what was the first case of a deaf person discriminated against at work because no adjustments were made to allow him to avoid telephone work.

Using a lipspeaker to help him understand the hearing, Mark won £7,436 in damages in this ground-breaking case.

He was interviewed for a job as a part-time medical records clerk for Lincolnshire Hospital NHS Trust. His application was unsuccessful since he could not answer incoming calls. But an employment tribunal in Nottingham argued that the job could easily have been rearranged so that he did not have to answer the phone.

Lincolnshire Hospital NHS Trust was found to be in breach of section 6 of the DDA. Mark was placed at a 'substantial disadvantage in comparison with other non-disabled persons by reason of his hearing impairment'.

He said: 'There are serious employment barriers for deaf people. Employers should attend a disability awareness training course to understand these barriers.

'If a deaf person feels that he or she has been discriminated against, I would recommend approaching the DRC for support. I wonder how often I have lost out on opportunities for finding work due to employers' ignorance. The Hospital Trust will now have to review its equal opportunities policy and ensure that managers know their responsibilities.

'I feel sad that this had to happen but if it leads to more deaf people getting jobs, something good will have come out of it.'

**Case study**

Phil, 34, is a journalist who works as features editor on a local newspaper in Reading, Berkshire. Married with a young daughter, he has also worked as deputy editor of the *Baptist Times* newspaper.

First diagnosed with a hearing problem in childhood, he now has about half his hearing in his right ear and around 70% in the left one.

He admits: 'It took me a long time to come to terms with having this disability. But I haven't allowed my hearing problem to hold me back in any area of my life.

'There are ways around the challenges at work. Most colleagues know I have a difficulty and are supportive. Recorded messages and call centres on the phone in particular can be a problem, so someone will usually step in and help me.

'It's especially hard if I am talking to someone I've not spoken to before, so I don't know their voice. I had an angry reader on the line once and the fact that I couldn't hear them just made them ever angrier!

'I avoid the phone wherever possible and prefer dealing with people face-to-face. These days, having Skype, instant messaging and so on makes life much easier. I also have every confidence that developing technology will make things even easier in the future.

'I'm also involved in the Baptist Men's Movement, and that means quite a lot of travelling round, talking to groups and meeting new people. Sometimes it can be hard standing chatting in groups, but somehow I always seem to manage. You just get on with it.'

# Summing Up

- The DDA makes it illegal for any employer to discriminate against any member of staff who has a disability, including a sensory impairment such as a hearing loss, at any point during their working relationship with that employee.

- It's important to be open about your hearing loss from the outset and to tell your employer about it as soon as you are able.

- Things your employer could reasonably provide include a wide range of equipment, a sign language interpreter and a reliance of written rather than oral communication.

- The government's Access to Work scheme offers advice on making these adjustments in a workplace and financial help.

- There are many things you can do if your employer won't listen or make the right adjustments for you – remember, the law is on your side. However, look on an employment tribunal as a last resort, only to be used when all other avenues have been explored.

# Chapter Six

## Technology

### Hearing aids

If you haven't worn a hearing aid before, it's important that you don't expect miracles overnight. Like anything else that's new, wearing a hearing aid takes some getting used to and it won't restore hearing to normal levels, but it is almost certainly the single most important piece of hearing equipment which can improve your quality of life.

Understandably, many people feel self-conscious when wearing a hearing aid for the first time, and rather daunted by the prospect, but it's important to persevere. Ask friends, family, colleagues and others around you to be supportive as you (and they) are getting used to it. Remember, a hearing aid isn't a magic wand that will suddenly give you perfect hearing.

Almost all hearing aids these days are digital and worn behind the ear, with a plastic mould which fits inside the ear.

### Analogue vs digital hearing aids

Analogue and digital aids may look similar but they process sound using different kinds of technology and offer varying benefits. Both kinds come in different sizes and styles.

Analogue hearing aids use conventional electronics. A microphone picks up the sound which a receiver (a tiny loudspeaker) then amplifies.

'An online survey among hearing aid users found that 6 in 10 people considered their decision to use hearing aids easy once they realised they had a hearing loss. Nearly 90% reported that their hearing aids have made a positive difference in their lives.'

Hear-It AISBL.

With digital hearing aids, a minuscule computer processes sound, meaning the device can be programmed to suit your particular hearing loss. Some digital aids are pre-progammable for different situations. Others adjust automatically to cope with different environments.

If your hearing changes, digital aids are re-programmable so can be updated accordingly. Many also have directional microphones, allowing you to hear and focus on sounds coming from in front of you more easily.

## Open-fit hearing aids

These are now quite commonplace for milder and high frequency losses and are available on the NHS. Like a behind-the-ear aid, they sit on top of the ear but are smaller. The part which goes inside the ear does not fill it entirely, which means that low frequency sounds can pass naturally through the small tip. Equally, it relieves the pressure from sounds such as your own voice, coughing and chewing and so on, which can sound uncomfortably loud.

## Settings

Ask your audiologist to fully explain how your hearing aid works, as nearly all aids have different settings. You may, for example, have one for an induction loop, one to eliminate background noise and another for normal use. You will hear different numbers of beeps for each setting, and there is often also a setting which you can use to put your aid on standby so that it is turned off while still in your ear. This could be very useful on a noisy train, for example. Some aids also have a volume control, often in the form of a small wheel on the back of the hearing aid.

## Batteries

You need to be shown how to remove and replace batteries. Most hearing aids emit a succession of short beeps to indicate when a battery has run down.

At night, or if you are not wearing your hearing aid for a long time, you may want to disconnect it by leaving the battery compartment open. Take care when opening the battery compartment since batteries have a habit of dropping out all over the place.

Don't be afraid to tell the person you're with if you need to change your hearing aid battery. It's better than struggling on and not being able to hear. If you feel self-conscious, excuse yourself for a couple of minutes and put in the new batteries somewhere private.

## What can the NHS do?

The NHS provides hearing aids to everyone who needs them free of charge, but they remain their property. You should return your aid if you are leaving the UK for any length of time, or if you no longer use or need it.

You will also get free batteries through the NHS for as long as you need them. Batteries are widely available from audiology departments and many GP surgeries, and you can collect new ones without an appointment. Often batteries can be posted to you if you are unable to pick them up yourself.

You will be given a brown 'record book' at the same time as your hearing aid. This is a record of any changes audiology staff make to your hearing aid and when you receive batteries. Always bring your book with you to any appointments about your hearing aid.

Your hearing aids can be adjusted as your hearing changes and your earmoulds replaced as necessary. However, although your audiology service can repair or replace your aid for free if you lose or damage it, you may be charged if this was your fault or keeps happening. It is your responsibility to look after your hearing aid, to make sure you wear it and to keep your supply of batteries topped up. Remember, it's hard to know when batteries run down and it can happen very suddenly, so always carry spares with you.

## NHS or private?

You can also buy hearing aids privately at your own expense, it is entirely your choice if you wish to do this. However, with NHS hearing aids now using very up-to-date technology, including digital technology, hopefully you should find NHS provision more than adequate.

The NHS cannot repair privately bought aids, or help towards the cost of buying them. However, buying a private aid doesn't affect your entitlement to an NHS one, so you can have both at the same time.

'Once it's been decided that you need a hearing aid, your audiologist will take an impression of your ear canal by filling it with a soft putty-like substance. This is a completely painless procedure.'

## Getting your hearing aid fitted

Once it's been decided that you need a hearing aid, your audiologist will take an impression of your ear canal by filling it with a soft putty-like substance. This is a completely painless procedure.

The impression will then be sent off to a lab for your aid to be made. Around three weeks later, you will have an appointment to fit the aid itself. Your audiologist will use computer equipment to test that the volume and tonal quality of your aid are right for you.

## Wearing your aid

The aid itself just hooks around the ear once the mould is in place, so focus on fitting the mould correctly in your ear first. If it's not inserted properly, it could feel uncomfortable and you may get feedback, or whistling. Your audiologist will show you how to put in and take out your hearing aid when you begin using it.

## Listening to sounds

You should not wear your new hearing aid full-time to start off with, but build up use gradually by wearing it for short periods – perhaps hour-long bursts up to three times a day. Follow your audiologist's advice on getting started with your hearing aid.

Even the slightest sound can seem horribly magnified when you use a new hearing aid. So try it out in a room with plenty of soft furnishings which absorb rather than reflect sound. In the first instance, listen to everyday sounds like footsteps, a shutting door or a boiling kettle, see how these sound and take it from there.

If things still sound uncomfortably loud a few months after your aid is fitted, your audiologist will adjust it for you.

Don't worry if everything sounds unnaturally loud – the noise levels will soon adjust themselves and settle down as you get used to them. A hearing aid won't make your hearing worse, so don't worry if everything sounds disproportionately faint once you take your aid out.

## Listening to people

Listen to just one person to start off with, from just a few feet away. Once you're happy with one-to-one conversation, you're ready to try chatting to two or more people in a quiet room. Don't worry if it takes you a little while to do this.

You may still miss some of the conversation, but try and follow it and take part. Remind people that they shouldn't talk too fast.

To start off using a hearing aid for TV, watch something like the news where only one person is talking at once. Remember, you can get a loop system fitted if you still find TV hard to hear – and there are always subtitles – see chapter 7 for more information.

## Trying your hearing aid out and about

Once you're used to wearing your hearing aid at home, it's time for the wider world. Somewhere you already know well, such as your garden or street, could be a good starting point.

Only wear your hearing aid somewhere like a busy shopping centre or where there is noisy traffic once you are comfortable with using it. You may find things too loud otherwise.

At parties and other social situations, you still may not understand everything, so be prepared for that. Remember that plenty of people who have perfect hearing sometimes find parties hard as well. Meetings and lectures can also be tricky to follow at times – your aid may pick up loudly on distracting sounds such as whispering or papers being shuffled.

## Care and maintenance

It's not a bad idea to wipe your earmould each time you take it out of your ear. It helps to stop wax from building up and chemists sell anti-bacterial wipes for this.

Your audiology department should also give you a little brush for cleaning your earmould. This has a small hook on one end of it for picking out any bits of wax which have become stuck in the tubing of the earmould.

## Replacing tubing

The tubing on your hearing aid should be changed a couple of times a year before it becomes too hardened and brittle. This can usually be done at a drop-in hearing aid clinic if your local audiology department has one.

Your audiologist can also often give you an instruction leaflet if you prefer to put in the new tubing yourself.

## Washing the earmould

If you find wax is blocking your earmould and tubing, you may find you need to wash it at least every week. This is easily done, just ask your audiologist for some advice on what to use and how to do it.

## Common hearing aid problems and when to seek help

Here are some things to try if your aid doesn't appear to be functioning properly:

'Only wear your hearing aid somewhere like a busy shopping centre or where there is noisy traffic once you are comfortable with using it; you may find things too loud otherwise.'

- Ensure you haven't accidentally changed the setting to the 'T' switch, or another wrong setting.

- Ensure you haven't turned down the volume to its lowest level.

- Make sure that the battery hasn't run out, and that it is in your aid the right way round (there's usually a + sign on the battery and on the compartment which should be matched up).

- Ensure your mould hasn't become blocked with ear wax.

- Check if the tubing has split, or become squashed or twisted.

If you have gone through this checklist and your aid is still not working, visit your local hearing aid clinic. You should also visit it if:

- Your hearing aid suddenly sounds very different.

- The mould itself has splits or cracks in it.

- The tubing becomes loose or needs to be changed.

- Your earmould or the tube keep slipping away from your ear.

Other problems may need an individual audiologist's appointment rather than a visit to the drop-in hearing aid clinic.

# Loop systems

You may also find that loop systems, also known as T-coil or telecoil systems, can help you to hear better in some situations by reducing or eliminating background noise. Many people find these systems make all the difference.

Essentially, an induction loop is a cable which goes around a room. It receives its signal via a direct connection with another sound source. This may be a sound system, TV or a microphone in front of the speaker.

If you are sitting within the loop's area, you can then pick up the signal and switch your aid to the 'T' or loop programme. Then you can adjust the volume on your aid as you would normally.

Many public buildings, including post offices, banks, supermarkets, cinemas, theatres and places of worship, have loops installed. Look out for the sign shown below.

If your hearing loop system doesn't appear to be working, check that your aid is switched on and turned to the right setting. And don't be afraid to ask staff in a public building whether a loop system is available and switched on.

More information on loop systems at home is available from your local social services department. Your hearing therapist can also help by giving you a loop system to try out.

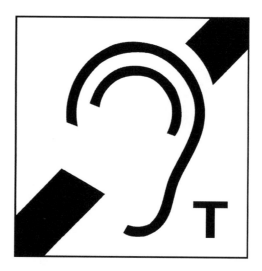

## Telephones, mobiles and textphones

Depending on the degree of your hearing loss, having a hearing problem doesn't necessarily mean you won't be able to communicate effectively on the telephone. That's not to say that phone conversations aren't sometimes challenging or frustrating, but modern technology now offers deaf people more choice than ever.

It's possible, for example, to buy telephones with built-in inductive couplers in the handset so that if you wear a hearing aid you can switch it to the 'T' setting, amplifying incoming sound.

Others have incoming and/or outgoing sound amplification or big buttons for easy dialling if the user has another disability such as arthritis or visual impairment. Some, designed with older people in mind, also have a button which connects directly to 999 services.

## Telephone amplifiers

As well as phones themselves, it's also possible to purchase telephone amplifiers to increase the volume of the caller's voice.

Clip-on amplifiers are both user-friendly and easy to install on any corded telephone.

In-line amplifiers fit between the handset and the base unit of the phone. The curly cable of the handset plugs into the amplifier, which you then connect to the base of the phone. You cannot use these amplifiers with cordless telephones, phones with numbers on the handset itself, or phones where the curly cable cannot be detached.

## Textphones

Text Relay is the national telephone relay service provided by BT, available 24 hours a day, every day. You do not pay extra for this service, and some phone companies even offer discounts on the text part of your call.

If you have a textphone, you can either type or speak the words you want to say. An operator can then relay this verbatim to the other person as simultaneous text, and the words appear on the screen. The other person can speak their response or type it on a keyboard. Textphones can also be used as an ordinary phone by hearing members of the household and often have a function to amplify incoming sound.

■ To use a textphone to call out, dial 18001 in front of the full phone number (using the STD code even if you are making a local call).

'Text Relay is the national telephone relay service provided by BT, available 24 hours a day, every day. You do not pay extra for this service, and some phone companies even offer discounts on the text part of your call.'

- If people want to call you on your textphone, they should prefix your full number with 18002.

## Mobile phones

Sending text messages is a great way to keep in touch if you find it hard to hear, especially when you're out and about, but having a hearing difficulty doesn't mean a complete end to talking on a mobile. In fact, the digital technology which mobile phones use means it can sometimes be easier to hear on a mobile than any other kind of phone.

A range of helpful mobiles is on offer, including:

- Phones with large buttons and screen if you have dexterity or sight problems.

- Voice amplification and good clarity.

- Phones which can be used with a hearing aid on a 'T' setting.

- Strong vibration to alert you to an incoming call.

---

**Case study**

Juliet's textphone

'At first I was wary of using a textphone, as it seemed a slightly daunting prospect. You have to overcome the psychological barrier of knowing that someone else is listening to your conversation, as do the people you are talking to. But the operators do a fantastic job and it's worth persevering with, even if it does take a bit of getting used to at first. Your friends, family and others you talk to regularly also have to adjust to this way of communicating and you need to be prepared for conversations to take a bit longer than normal. For me it's certainly less frustrating than battling on with a standard phone.

'I have one friend who I chat to a lot on the phone and at times it was very frustrating all round trying to communicate. Now we can jabber away all evening if we want to. The textphone has saved a lot of frustration all round.'

---

## Mobile accessories

Mobile phones sometimes cause interference with hearing aids. For that reason, you may find accessories like neckloops and ear hooks helpful because they increase the distance between your aid and your phone, reducing the risk of feedback and interference.

# Other equipment

As well as hearing aids and all kinds of telephones, a wide range of other equipment is available to help people who are deaf or hard of hearing. This includes flashing doorbells, vibrating alarm clocks and watches and special baby and smoke alarms.

## Listening equipment

You can also buy a variety of other mobile listening equipment to help you hear conversations, TV, radio or music. Some personal listeners are suitable for milder hearing losses, and some (but not all) are designed to be used with hearing aids.

Many listening products can be worn with headphones, stethoclips or earbuds. Some also come with a neckloop or ear hooks so that hearing aid wearers can use them with their aid on a 'T' setting.

RNID offers a wide range of equipment through its catalogue. Visit www.rnid. org.uk/shop to see a range of their products.

## Skype

Skype is free of charge and available via the Internet. The company may try and sell you headphones and other accessories but you don't have to buy them. It allows you to have typed instant message conversations with anyone else in the world who has Skype, or speak to them for free on Skype using a webcam to enable lipreading.

Most of the main Internet Service Providers and Facebook also have instant messaging functions, while Microsoft Communicator is part of Microsoft Office and offers a similar service.

# Summing Up

▪ Hearing aids are not miracle cures, and they take some getting used to. They come as analogue, digital, behind-the-ear or open-fit models.

▪ Wearing an aid can take persistence and perseverance, both for you and those around you. Build up your use gradually.

▪ You will need to learn about the various settings and care and maintenance of your aid, but all of these are quite straightforward.

▪ Although private provision is available, you should find NHS aids, which now include digital models, to be more than adequate.

▪ Specially adapted mobile and landline phones and textphones all make telephone conversations a real possibility for deaf and hard of hearing people.

▪ Instant messaging and mobile phone texting give you other communication options.

▪ Other equipment is available to help you enjoy the radio, TV or music, and to hear your alarm clock or smoke alarm.

# Chapter Seven

# Communication

## TV subtitles and signed programmes

For many deaf or hearing impaired people, whatever the level of their loss, subtitles offer the perfect way to watch and follow TV while keeping volumes at unobtrusive levels. It is now a legal obligation for the most popular channels (of which there were 78 in 2009) to subtitle a certain percentage of their output. Most exceed these minimum statutory quotas.

TV channels also have to provide signed programmes and audio description for the blind or visually impaired, but subtitling is by far the largest of these.

### TV subtitles

As well as word-for-word dialogue, subtitles are a textual representation of sound effects like laughter or applause, or a description of background music. Different speakers' words are usually relayed in separate colours.

The extent to which you rely on subtitles will depend on the degree of your hearing loss, your age and levels of literacy. For some people, subtitles are just useful as a back-up reference for the odd missed word. Others rely on subtitles completely.

More than 70 channels were required to provide access services this year. Most of these had to subtitle at least 60% of their programming this year, with the BBC's target much higher, at 100% for all its output.

In the third quarter of 2009, all the main terrestrial channels subtitled at least 80% of their programmes. These statistics all represent a huge leap forward from the rather patchy subtitling services provided even just a few years ago.

'The extent to which you rely on subtitles will depend on the degree of your hearing loss, your age and levels of literacy. For some people, subtitles are just useful as a back-up reference for the odd missed word. Others rely on subtitles completely.'

## Signed TV programmes

All the main terrestrial TV stations must also provide signing on at least 5% of their programmes. In 2009, nine of the other larger digital channels were also required to provide some level of signed programming. Again, all these targets were exceeded in the third quarter of 2009. There are 62 channels with small audiences who are obliged to either show 30 minutes of sign-presented programming or pay into a fund that makes sign-presented programming for broadcast during the Community Channel's dedicated BSL Zone.

Signed programmes have been a feature of public service TV for some years. Most of these are sign-interpreted versions of programmes made for hearing people, rather than sign-presented programming made specifically for people with a hearing impairment. It is up to the broadcaster to decide which programmes to sign and when to schedule them.

Signed programmes may be especially helpful for the profoundly deaf, who tend to find fast or complex subtitles especially hard to follow.

# How subtitling works

The recommended font for subtitles is Tiresias Screenfont, designed for subtitling on UK digital television in 1998.

In the past, subtitles were called up using Teletext page 888. Now subtitles are displayed digitally, or as though they were digital. If you haven't yet switched to digital TV, you can still access subtitles via your TV remote on page 888.

This service will continue to be available until the digital switchover takes place in your region – all regions will be switched over by the end of 2012. If you have already switched to digital television, you should find that the subtitles are clearer and easier to read. They are also more consistently accurate.

If you have a set-top box as most satellite, cable and Freeview viewers do, you can use its remote control to call up the subtitles instead.

Independent subtitling companies such as Red Bee Media are commissioned by broadcasters to produce the subtitles for their programmes. Subtitles for live programmes are generated either by stenographers or by individuals trained in using voice recognition software.

Inevitably, with some live programmes such as news reports, the subtitling can sometimes be inaccurate. Equally, with live programmes a short delay in transmission is inevitable, given the time it takes to generate subtitles.

## DVD subtitles

Look at the DVD box to see whether a film can be played with subtitles. You may find the film has subtitles in other languages, straight English subtitles and subtitles for the deaf and hard of hearing which include descriptions of noises as well as speech.

Google has recently announced that it will be developing software so that more videos can be subtitled on websites such as YouTube.

## Cinema subtitling

Of course, at one time all films had captions! But since the long-gone era of silent movies, with the exception of foreign language pictures, deaf and hard of hearing people have routinely found cinema trips extremely difficult.

Happily, things are changing, and it's more possible to see subtitled movies in a cinema than it has ever been. This is largely thanks to technological developments, such as 'open' subtitling which allows cinemas to project captions directly onto the screen during the showing of a standard release copy of the film. This is more flexible. Previously, cinemas showed 'hard' captioned copies of movies, with the captions already overlaid. Often, screenings of these versions took place at unsociable times such as Sunday mornings.

## Theatre captioning

STAGETEXT is a registered charity which provides captioning services to theatres that want to make their productions accessible to deaf, deafened and hard of hearing people.

**Case study**

Ian's story

'I finally got a chance to see *Slumdog Millionaire*. I bought some popcorn, met my friend, settled down, lights dimmed, film started. And then what happened? No subtitles.

'I was furious. My hearing friend for a deaf person, Catherine, went out to make enquiries and was told that the projector wasn't working. Catherine told me that she had the distinct impression someone had just forgotten to turn the subtitles on. After about five minutes, the subtitles finally came on.

'It was only five minutes, and I stayed to enjoy the rest of the film. But it didn't alleviate my fury. It's just not good enough.'

Captions are similar to television subtitles but include additional information, such as indications of characters' names, sound effects, offstage noises and musical descriptions. The actors' words appear on an LED display unit (or units) placed next to the stage or in the set at the same time as they are spoken or sung.

A trained captioner prepares everything in advance, working closely with the production team, then operates the captions as the action unfolds on stage.

Many theatres now provide captioning services in-house and use local captioners who have been trained by STAGETEXT.

STAGETEXT sometimes also uses a speech-to-text reporter for talks or discussions with the director and cast members following a captioned performance. On these occasions, the dialogue also appears on the caption unit, enabling everyone to ask questions and play a full part in the discussion.

# Speech-to-text transcription

Speech-to-text transcription enables deaf, deafened and hard of hearing people to follow and participate fully in work and educational settings, live public lectures and discussions where the text is not prepared in advance.

A highly trained speech-to-text reporter (STTR) uses a special phonetic keyboard which converts everything into English, using systems called Palantype and Stenograph. STTRs work at high speeds and produce speech verbatim.

## Tips for enjoying theatre, films and concerts

- If you use a hearing loop, try to pre-book tickets for seats where the loop will be most effective, or as near the front of the hall or as close to loudspeakers as possible.

- You may want to turn down your hearing aid, if you wear one, at the end of a performance, as loud applause can sound quite uncomfortable.

# Communication tips and strategies

There are many practical things you can do to make conversation easier all round if you have a hearing problem. Here are some suggestions:

## Be open

Admittedly, this isn't always an easy one. But, if possible, it's usually a good idea to explain that you have a hearing problem. People are generally then much more willing to help and understand. Never feel embarrassed or ashamed to explain that you can't hear. Be factual and open in your explanation and be prepared for questions – people will probably want to know the cause and when you first started to lose your hearing.

'Sub-titled films and captioned theatre plays are wonderful, and have opened up a whole new world of entertainment for me and many other deaf and hard of hearing people.'

Laetitia.

## Make sure the speaker has your attention

If the speaker doesn't have your attention when they begin talking to you, you may well miss the first words they say which can get the whole conversation off to a tricky start.

Stand or sit as close as comfortably possible to the speaker or other sound source, and turn your better ear (if you have one) towards them. Ask people to try and remember to talk to you on your 'best' side, if you have one, and stand on the 'right' side of you.

Also, explain to people you will not be able to hear them if they say something while they are walking away from you.

## What the speaker can do

If you don't have a 'best' side, ask the speaker to face you, as this allows you to watch their lips and follow their facial expressions and gestures. Ask the person you are talking to not to cover their mouth or chew while they are speaking to you.

You might hear better in a well-lit room as people's faces will be lit-up – you have every right to ask for this, for example if you are attending a job interview.

Ask people not to speak to you or to approach you from behind, as this can make you jump.

## Louder isn't better

Unfortunately, many people simply increase the volume when they are talking to someone with a hearing loss, but this rarely helps. Instead, ask people to speak to you more clearly and slowly and without exaggerating sounds.

## It does matter!

Try not to let someone get away with saying 'It doesn't matter'. This can be infuriating. After all, if something doesn't matter, why have they mentioned it in the first place?

In these situations, it's a personal decision as to how long you want to persist in asking people to repeat themselves. You could use humour, charm or cajoling, but do try and get them to understand that repeating what you have missed is the right thing to do.

## If you don't hear

If you haven't heard someone, there are things you can do which may help. You can ask the speaker to rephrase rather than simply repeat what they have said. If you miss a key word or phrase, such as a surname or place name and you don't get it after several repetitions, ask them to write it down.

If you're not sure whether you've heard correctly, repeat it back as you have understood it, and ask them to confirm you have understood properly.

## Don't bluff

It can be tempting to smile and nod or say something non-committal if you haven't heard. But if you try and bluff your way through a conversation, you could just end up adding to the confusion. So it's best not to pretend to understand if you haven't. You shouldn't be afraid to look puzzled if you haven't heard – a good communicator will pick up on this and clarify what they have said very quickly.

## Interruptions

Of course, in conversations people interrupt each other all the time. But sometimes, if you are in a group, you may find yourself talking over someone else simply because you haven't heard them speaking. So, if you realise you have done this, just explain that you didn't hear them talking and invite them to finish what they were saying.

## Keep calm

It's easy to become flustered if you think you have missed something. But the more you panic, or the longer you reflect and wonder what you might have missed, the harder it becomes to rejoin the flow of the conversation.

'If you don't hear someone, there are things you can do which may help. You can ask the speaker to rephrase rather than simply repeat what they have said. If you miss a key word or phrase, such as a surname or place name and you don't get it after several repetitions, ask them to write it down.'

# Tips and strategies for out and about

### Public transport

This can sometimes be quite tricky, although certainly not impossible. If buying a ticket through a glass screen, ask whether a hearing loop can be switched on. Most airports and stations provide information on screens, but you may miss tannoy announcements, especially on railway platforms. If no one is travelling with you, don't be afraid to ask strangers to repeat announcements for you.

### Shopping and eating out

Shops, cafes and restaurants can often be noisy places. You will learn to develop coping strategies and how to guess the question you're being asked. For example, if you're ordering a coffee or tea, you'll probably be asked about milk and sugar. You can ask restaurants to turn background music down (surveys have shown that most people are indifferent to it anyway) and sit away from speakers.

Hearing Concern Link has a badge scheme to let shop assistants know that someone is deaf, hard of hearing or a lipreader (see help list for details).

## The right listening environment

- You can help create a better environment for listening by eliminating background noise such as radio or TV. You can also shut windows and doors to eliminate sound like traffic which cannot be turned down.

- Let others know you won't be able to hear if they talk or call out to you from another room, and, equally, do not expect to be able to hear anyone who is talking in another room.

- If you sit with your back against a wall, this will help to reduce background noise and reflect noise back towards you.

- If you are using a loop system, check that it is working properly, and report it if it isn't.

- At home, soft furnishings such as thick carpets and heavy curtains, as well as double-glazing, will help create a better listening environment for you, since sound reverberates off hard surfaces.

# British Sign Language

BSL is the most commonly used sign language in the UK, and is a way of communicating using gestures, facial expressions and body language. In fact, it's a beautiful language!

Since March 2003, BSL has enjoyed government recognition as a minority language. For up to 70,000 people across Britain, it is the language in which they prefer to communicate.

BSL has its own grammar, syntax and word order, and is not particularly closely linked to spoken English.

It's a common misconception that the same sign language is used across the world, but that's just not the case. There are even great differences within BSL in different British regions, just as there are varied accents in spoken language. In fact, there can even be variations from town to town, such as the Manchester system of number signs, for example.

Other countries have their own kinds of sign language and these bear no relation to BSL. In America, for example, US sign language is very different to BSL, even though English is the main spoken language.

Under the Police and Criminal Evidence Act 1984 and the DDA 1995, deaf and hard of hearing people are entitled to BSL interpreters in some situations.

'Since March 2003, BSL has enjoyed government recognition as a minority language. For up to 70,000 people across Britain, it is the language in which they prefer to communicate.'

## Learning BSL

You can learn BSL at evening classes at local colleges, deaf centres and some private organisations. You can also learn online through an organisation such as www.british-sign.co.uk.

The Qualifications and Curriculum Development Agency (QCDA) provides awards at the following levels:

- Level I – Elementary.
- Level II – Intermediate.
- Level III/ NVQ 3 – Advanced.
- NVQ 4 – Required as part of the NVQ 4 BSL/English Interpreting.

The British Deaf Association has formed the BSL Academy, providing an official British Sign Language curriculum and tutor training.

## Sign Supported English

Sign Supported English (SSE) is another kind of sign language found in the UK. Although it isn't actually a language in itself, it uses BSL signs – but in the same word order as spoken English.

SSE is most commonly used as a way of supporting oral English, particularly in schools where children are learning English grammar at the same time as BSL.

## Fingerspelling

Fingerspelling is a communication method which uses hand movements to spell out words.

In BSL, it can be used to spell out a name or place for which there is no official sign, or if there is some confusion and someone doesn't understand a particular sign. There is one fingerspelling sign for each letter of the alphabet.

Some aspects of fingerspelling are also incorporated into individual BSL signs.

However, using fingerspelling to hold a conversation would take too long and would not bring the same level of feeling and expression as sign language would.

Learning to fingerspell is easy and free, visit www.british-sign.co.uk.

# Lipreading

Lipreading, sometimes also known as speechreading, is the ability to recognise different speech sounds by observing different movements of the lips, tongue and jaws. The shape of the lips remains fractionally after the sound of a word has disappeared, giving you slightly more time to lipread than if you hear with your ears alone.

Effectively, with lipreading your eyes become your ears. It is a huge help to millions of people in the UK with a hearing problem, especially those who were not born deaf.

It's not a perfect way to communicate – many sounds in the English language cannot be detected just by seeing them on the speaker's lips, and sounds made in the back of the throat cannot be heard at all. So other clues are needed, such as context or facial expression, to understand what has been said. You only have to see the sounds of the letters 'p' and 'b', for example, to see that they look the same.

Bits of conversation which appear in isolation or without supporting information, such as the name of someone you've never met before, can also be easy to miss if you are relying on lipreading alone.

Lipreading tends to work best when also used in conjunction with other help such as a strong hearing aid, fingerspelling or sign language.

## What are the best lipreading conditions?

■ Ideally, hold one-to-one conversations where possible.

■ If you are in a group, only speak to one person at a time.

■ Make sure there is plenty of light on the speaker's face.

■ Ask the speaker not to turn away.

■ Obstructions such as hands over the mouth are an obvious hindrance.

■ Beards and moustaches also make lipreading difficult.

■ Lipreading involves looking at the whole face – you need to be able to see the speaker's eyes as well.

- Holding a conversation in a room like a kitchen, where there tend to be lots of hard surfaces and noisy equipment, can also make lipreading more challenging.

- Lipreading through a glass screen can be difficult. If you need to have a long conversation in a bank or somewhere similar, ask for a private conversation in a quiet room without a screen.

## Learning lipreading

While many people with a hearing loss lipread almost without realising they are doing it, a class will help you develop and practice this skill. Lipreading is taught to adults in local colleges, community centres and at hard of hearing clubs across the UK.

The emphasis is on informality – there are no exams or qualifications. While some teachers will hold classes for different levels of lipreading students, in general classes tend to be of mixed ability. The subject is taught phonetically, so that you learn shapes of the mouth by how they sound.

Teachers train through the Association of Teachers of Lipreading to Adults (ATLA), who can give you information about a class in your area.

Irene, a lipreading teacher from Hampshire, has 17 years of experience teaching lipreading and takes classes across the south of England. She says: 'For people who may be losing their hearing, it's a good idea to come while they still have some hearing left. That way, they will gain more from the classes.

'Many students find that, as well as mastering the skill, there are huge social benefits. They find an environment where they feel comfortable, and find empathy with like minded people. We all have a lot of fun, and it's lovely to see people's confidence grow. The great thing is that no one ever feels left out.'

# Lipspeaking

A lipspeaker is a trained professional who is easy to lipread. They can be booked to provide access to communication for someone who is deaf or hearing impaired, for example, at a hospital appointment and in legal, educational and other settings.

'When you are deaf you live inside a well-corked glass bottle. You see the entrancing outside world, but it does not reach you. After learning to lip read, you are still inside the bottle, but the cork has come out and the outside world slowly but surely comes in to you.'

Dorothy Clegg, author of *The Listening Eye.*

Lipspeakers repeat clearly everything that has been said, moving their lips without sound and using the flow, rhythm and phrasing of natural speech. The lipspeaker will use appropriate gestures, facial expression and fingerspelling where necessary to help understanding. They are never more than a sentence behind the speaker. If necessary and appropriate, lipspeakers can also use their voice to help the lipreading process and provide a voiced transmission of the lipreader's message.

There is always a slight delay from what is being said. Although voicing can be used if the client wishes, in conferences and some other situations this is not always appropriate.

It's a very small profession, with fewer than 100 certificated and registered lipspeakers in the UK. It's also a 'young' organisation, having only been devised in 1948.

If you are deaf or hearing impaired, you have the same right to book a lipspeaker as you would a sign language interpreter. For almost all situations, the cost of using a professional lipspeaker is met by the service provider, not the lipreader. If you are in employment, the cost of lipspeaker provision is paid for through the Access to Work fund.

A wide range of communication support for a variety of situations is available through RNID. This includes:

- BSL interpreters.
- Lipspeakers.
- Speech-to-text reporters.
- Deafblind interpreters.
- Communciation support workers.
- Note-takers.
- Video interpreters.

To book, visit RNID's website or get in touch with your regional RNID communication support office (see help list).

# Summing Up

■ TV subtitles allow you to follow programmes without turning the volume up and are a wonderful help for many deaf and hard of hearing people. TV channels are required to provide a set amount of subtitled and signed programmes in their yearly output.

■ It's also possible to watch subtitled DVDs and, increasingly, films in the cinema.

■ Captioning services are available for some stage productions and other public events.

■ There are many strategies to aid communication – learn what works best for you.

■ Lipreading classes are sociable, fun and incredibly helpful. Start to learn to lipread sooner rather than later.

■ Sign language and fingerspelling are popular communication methods for those with severe or profound deafness.

■ Lipspeakers are professionals who are trained to be easily lipread and can help in many situations where good understanding is essential, such as court cases or hospital appointments.

Need2Know

# Chapter Eight

# Tinnitus

## What is tinnitus?

Tinnitus comes from the Latin word for 'ringing' and is the name given to the condition in which noises are heard despite there being no external source. People who have tinnitus say it sounds like ringing, whistling, buzzing or humming.

Diagnosis is generally by people describing their symptoms. There is no specific medication or operation to cure it. Instead there are various approaches patients can try to tackle the problem.

Tinnitus occurs across all age groups and even quite young children can experience it, so it is not accurately described as a condition exclusive to older people.

Around 1 in 10 of the population experiences mild tinnitus at some point in their lives, and up to 1% of adults with tinnitus may find it's severe enough to affect their quality of life.

The pitch varies – sounds can have a high, medium or low pitch, and the noises may be heard in one or both ears or in the middle of the head. Equally, it may sometimes be difficult to pinpoint the sound's exact location.

Many people who have tinnitus do not find it an upsetting or invasive condition. For others, however, its onset can cause distress.

# Causes of tinnitus

The exact causes of tinnitus are still not entirely understood, although it is known that the symptoms are generated within the sufferer's auditory pathways. There is a strong link between tinnitus and some kinds of hearing loss.

Tinnitus should not be considered as an illness, nor is it caused by any disease of the ears.

There may be several underlying reasons behind tinnitus development, and, for some people, its onset follows a stressful event, either physical or emotional, such as bereavement or a head injury. It can also be particularly prevalent following exposure to loud noise.

'The exact causes of tinnitus are still not entirely understood, although it is known that the symptoms are generated within the sufferer's auditory pathways.'

# Sudden onset tinnitus

Where there is a trigger such as a stressful event or a head injury and tinnitus comes about suddenly, this can lead to unfounded fears of a very serious condition such as a brain tumour. Unfortunately, this worry often just increases the brain's awareness of the tinnitus, creating a vicious circle and making things worse.

# Auditory memory and tinnitus

The brain analyses and stores useful information about useful sounds such as speech, but it also throws out sounds that are not needed by a process of rejection known as filtration.

What happens sometimes is that this process can fail, which leads to an unwanted sound being perceived in the cerebral cortex area of the brain. This can form the basis of tinnitus generation.

Equally, the brain also has the ability to increase its awareness of sound – known as auditory gain. This can happen in different situations, for example:

- If someone is under stress.

- In a place where there is total silence, in which case the brain becomes aware of random activity in the hearing pathway which the filtration process would generally reject.

# Managing tinnitus

It's a common misconception that if you have tinnitus, nothing can be done to cure it or alleviate the symptoms. In fact, there are many things you can try to manage this condition.

If you have tinnitus, tinnitus retraining therapy may be carried out by a doctor, a hearing therapist, an audiological scientist or audiologist and may include one or more of the kinds of things listed below.

- Relaxation – simple relaxation techniques can be very helpful in managing tinnitus, by recognising and controlling tension.

- Diet and drink – while some people find alcohol or foods like cheese can aggravate their tinnitus, other people find the very same things actually make it better. So people's responses are very individual, and the only way to know whether something will work for you is to remove it from your diet then reintroduce it to assess what affect it has on your tinnitus.

- Medication – the number of drugs with a genuine link to tinnitus is actually very small. However, there is a very small group of drugs which can cause tinnitus. Mainly, these medications are prescribed in cases of serious illness, generally when there is no alternative.

- Tinnitus management devices – to manage their tinnitus, many people find it helpful to use a device providing constant low-level noise which is lower than the level of the tinnitus. The advantage of a low-level noise device is that it can retrain the brain to ignore meaningless sound, which will slowly reduce the focus on the tinnitus.

- Support groups – many people with tinnitus find support groups invaluable. Such groups can be a great way of meeting new friends, sharing ideas about tinnitus management and reminding yourself that you are not alone.

'It's a common misconception that if you have tinnitus, nothing can be done to cure it or alleviate the symptoms. In fact, there are many things you can try to manage this condition.'

# Tinnitus and complementary therapies

Some people, dissatisfied with the symptom-focused approach of their GPs, want to play a more active role in their treatment, and turn to complementary therapies. We are still quite uninformed about the effectiveness of complementary therapy in general, and those for tinnitus in particular.

- Gingko Biloba is a herbal supplement available in health food shops and derives from the Chinese Maidenhair tree. Three quite small studies carried out in the 1990s showed Gingko to be fairly effective in reducing tinnitus, but the largest study carried out to date showed more disappointing results. A team at Birmingham University concluded that Gingko was not an effective treatment for tinnitus for most people, although certain individuals might benefit.

- Acupuncture – a study in 1998 showed some improvements in tinnitus for 45% of patients following acupuncture but these improvements did not last. Another six studies showed no positive effect.

- Homeopathy – so far only one study has been carried out into tinnitus and homeopathy, and this showed that the homeopathic remedy had no effect.

- Many other forms of complementary therapy are recommended for tinnitus, amongst them zinc supplements, vitamin B and restricted diets. But, as yet, not enough scientific evidence exists to make any judgements about whether they are effective or not, although plenty of anecdotal evidence does exist.

Compared to many forms of conventional medicine, most complementary therapies are very safe. But side effects from herbal medicines are possible – people have reported headaches and stomach upsets after taking Gingko Biloba, and there can also be negative health effects caused by large doses of vitamin and mineral supplements.

For many, having tinnitus means more than hearing an internal noise. It means feeling anxious, getting depressed or not being able to sleep. It is well proven that people feel more able to get on top of their tinnitus when they are feeling otherwise well in themselves. For some, complementary therapy may be a way of reaching a sense of improved wellbeing, so they may be an option for those who are struggling with other problems surrounding their tinnitus.

The placebo effect is strong in many complementary therapy trials, including those for tinnitus. This means that in many of the studies where treatment was shown to be ineffective, a number of people did experience improvements in their tinnitus. It was just that a similar number of people responded to the placebo treatment.

If you are considering complementary therapy for tinnitus, arm yourself with as much information as possible. Consider the potential dangers and be aware of the lack of any real evidence to date.

## Childhood tinnitus

As we mentioned earlier, it is possible to have tinnitus in childhood and the condition is equally common across all age groups. However, it is rare for it to persist into adulthood.

Tinnitus is common in children with a hearing impairment, and a child who has had tinnitus for a while may consider the situation 'normal' and so not complain about it.

The first step is to discuss the situation with your GP, who may make a referral to an ENT consultant.

Here are some of the things you could do to help your child:

- Reassurance – many children with tinnitus feel they are the only person to experience it. They may be concerned there may be a serious underlying reason for the symptom.

- Explanation – a young child may need a simpler explanation than an adult.

- Hope – offer hope that this condition will not last forever.

- Sound generators – as described above.

- Avoidance of quietness – most patients with tinnitus notice the symptom is worse in quiet surroundings.

- Relaxation – if tinnitus is worsened by stress, for example at exam time, relaxation techniques could well help.

- Further help could also be useful, for example from a psychologist.

## Case study

Helen, 40, from Cardiff, is a deputy supervisor in a police non-emergency contact centre. She has been experiencing tinnitus for around 18 years, but it was not recognised for the first three of these.

Helen hears a dull droning noise in one ear and a hissing noise in both. She says:

'At first I was told I was imagining it, then that I was experiencing this because I was stressed. My original doctor had no understanding, left me feeling awful and didn't give me any useful information.

'I went online, found the British Tinnitus Association and discovered that the University of Wales Hospital had a dedicated unit dealing with tinnitus. I asked to be referred there and they ran tests which confirmed that my hearing was good, but it was tinnitus which was making me think I was going deaf.

'It can affect my working life sometimes. It also means I can't go to pubs, clubs, gigs or anywhere else where the noise is above a certain level, or where there will be very loud music.

'I've taught myself to deal with it as best I can. I find that complete silence makes things worse so I put a radio on or play music quietly in the background to try to hide the noise. I miss not being able to have complete silence. When it's bad, sometimes I withdraw into myself.

'Luckily it hasn't affected family life too much, although now my mum has it and so I have helped her to cope. Sometimes, you just need someone who has experienced tinnitus to talk to.

'I would encourage anyone with tinnitus to keep on at their doctor for help, and to ask the British Tinnitus Association for advice.'

Need2Know

# Summing Up

- If you have tinnitus, you will 'hear' sounds even though there is no external source. It is not an illness.

- Tinnitus can affect children as well as adults.

- The causes of this condition are poorly understood, although it can follow an emotional, psychological or physical event.

- There is a definite link between tinnitus and some kinds of hearing loss.

- It's wrong to think you can do nothing about tinnitus – it can be managed with relaxation techniques, attendance at support groups and management devices which produce a low-level sound.

- For some people, switching certain drinks or foods can have an effect on their tinnitus.

- Very few medications are thought to have some connection with tinnitus, but never alter anything you have been prescribed without talking to your GP first.

- A wide range of complementary treatments, from acupuncture to herbal supplements, are available. But there is little hard evidence that they really work, and some alternative treatments can be very expensive.

# Chapter Nine

# Cochlear Implants

Sometimes called 'bionic ears', cochlear implants are electronic devices which are surgically inserted under a general anaesthetic to help people who are severely or profoundly deaf. The implant helps the wearer to hear speech as well as other sounds. It works by electrically stimulating the auditory nerve.

Most deaf people in the UK have sensorineural hearing loss (as described in chapter 1) and so have damaged cochlear hair cells. Implants are able to bypass these damaged cells and stimulate the auditory nerve directly.

Implants work best when someone has already had some language before losing their hearing and for young children who were born deaf. While the sounds may not be just as the person remembered them, they become more meaningful and natural with training and as the wearer grows used to their implant.

However, just as with hearing aids, they should not be viewed as a miracle cure. The sounds picked up by someone wearing a cochlear implant are not the same as those heard by the human ear.

By April 2009, there were nearly 190,000 users of cochlear implants worldwide. This was mainly in developed countries, given the high cost of the procedure to fit the implants, as well as the expense of the devices themselves and the post-surgical care. Only a fraction – around 6,000 – have implants in both ears, but this number is growing all the time.

'Sometimes called "bionic ears", cochlear implants are electronic devices which are surgically inserted under a general anaesthetic to help people who are severely or profoundly deaf.'

# UK cochlear implant wearers: facts and figures

- In Britain today, there are some 7,000 users of cochlear implants.

- In 2007, more than 350 adults and 430 children were implanted.

- Total cost for adult cochlear implantation, over a projected 30 years of use, is around £44,000. For children, the figure is higher given that they need more rehabilitation and training to get used to an implant.

# What does an implant look like? How does it work?

A cochlear implant consists of two parts:

- A processor – worn externally, including a microphone and transmitter coil.

- An implant – implanted beneath the skin.

The microphone picks up the sounds which the sophisticated speech processor converts to digitally coded signals which are transmitted to the internal implant as radio waves.

The implant interprets the signals into specialised patterns of electrical current which are sent down the electrode to the cochlea. These electrical pulses stimulate the auditory nerve which then sends this message to the brain for processing.

## 'Ear level' and 'body worn' processors

While an ear-level processor looks like a behind-the-ear hearing aid and is worn like one, body-worn processors are small boxes, attached to a belt or slipped into a pocket. Most users prefer behind-the-ear processors, as they are smaller and many people think they look better. However, for some users, it is more suitable for them to have a body-worn processor.

# Being assessed for an implant

Assessment for suitability for cochlear implants is carried out on an individual basis. Crucially, you must be fit and healthy enough to withstand the surgery.

Britain has around 20 implant centres. If you would like to explore the possibility of cochlear implantation, your first step should be to talk to your GP. Both children and adults undergo a thorough assessment first.

The assessment may include medical examinations, interviews and questionnaires. It will look at many things including:

- Your hearing.
- Speech and lipreading skills.
- Lifestyle.
- General health.
- What you expect to achieve by having a cochlear implant.

## The decision to undergo surgery

The implant team makes the recommendation that someone is a suitable candidate, but the ultimate decision is always down to the individual, or, in the case of children, the family.

The surgery is not reversible and implantation of the electrode in the cochlea usually destroys any residual hearing, meaning it is not possible to go back to using a hearing aid. The potential loss of any residual hearing, which is often very limited even with a hearing aid, must be weighed up against the potential to hear better with an implant.

## Having an implant fitted

The internal parts can only be surgically fitted under a general anaesthetic. You may have to stay in hospital for a night or two and the operation will usually take between two and four hours.

A month or six weeks afterwards, the 'switch on' takes place. This means that the speech processor is activated and programmed for individual use. You can also expect a period of extensive training and testing to maximise the benefit of wearing the device.

## What happens next?

Although you could choose not to wear the external part of the equipment later in life if you have an implant fitted as a child, few people decide to do this.

Both children and adults need yearly check-ups for their cochlear implants for the first few years of having them. After this, when everything is stable, the wearer can report any problems with the equipment and will only need to see the hospital if there is a problem.

## Children and cochlear implant surgery

Most children now are implanted between the age of one and two, so there isn't a lot parents can do to prepare their child, although the ward nurses work hard to make the situation comfortable. Most ENT wards that take children for implants have a nominated nurse who has at least level one sign language.

Only a few children need to stay overnight, but usually parents can stay with the child throughout.

## Deaf politics and cochlear implantation

People within the Deaf community describe themselves as Deaf with a capital D, and identify themselves as being culturally and politically, as well as physically, deaf.

As explained earlier, these members of the Deaf community see BSL as their first language and oppose any perceived attempts to suppress it. For the same reason, some Deaf parents do not want their children to have cochlear implants fitted.

'The internal parts can only be surgically fitted under a general anaesthetic. You may have to stay in hospital for a night or two and the operation will usually take between two and four hours.'

There has also been some resistance to cochlear implants from members of the Deaf community who feel that a young child whose own views are not being sought should not be subjected to this invasive surgery.

At the same time, some Deaf parents have not wanted hearing loss treated as a medical problem. Rather, Deaf people see themselves as part of a cultural minority.

Equally, there has been some concern about the unknown long-term effects of implantation, and there are fears for the future of the signing deaf population if implants allow children to grow up without the need for sign language. All these concerns influenced some parents in the early days of cochlear implantation.

Unsurprisingly, this is a controversial and highly sensitive area and one which continues to give rise to strong feelings on both sides of the debate.

However, now the benefits are better understood, most hearing parents of deaf children do opt for an implant if it is suggested, although Deaf parents of deaf children may still prefer not to implant their children.

# NICE recommendations

NICE produces guidance on public health, health technologies such as new medicines and drugs, and clinical practice. Once NICE guidance is published, health professionals are expected to take it fully into account when deciding what treatments to give people. In January 2009, NICE published technology appraisal guidance on cochlear implants for children and adults with severe to profound deafness.

This recommends a cochlear implant in one ear if you have severe to profound deafness, do not get enough benefit from hearing aids after trying them for three months and the cochlear implant team thinks you would benefit from an implant.

If you are a child or you are an adult who is blind or has another disability which means you rely on hearing sounds for spatial awareness, you should be able to have cochlear implants in both ears if these are placed in the same operation. If you already had an implant in one ear when the guidance was published, you should have the option of an additional contralateral implant only if this is considered likely to provide sufficient benefit by your cochlear implant team.

To read the guidance in full, visit www.nice.org.uk/TA166. If you think you are eligible for treatment but it is not available, see www.nice.org.uk/aboutguidance.

---

## Case study

Jamie's story

Lisa, 33, lives with her husband Dave, 34, in East Yorkshire. They have a hearing daughter called Mikyla, nine, and a severely hearing impaired son Jamie, now two and a half. Jamie had a cochlear implant operation when he was 19 months old, and Lisa and Dave now run an online support group for parents of children who may need cochlear implants.

Lisa says: 'We lost Dave's dad about eight weeks before Jamie was born, so were already under a lot of stress. We were told Jamie had a severe/profound loss at four weeks and it felt as though our whole world had fallen apart. Despite the tests, they never found a reason for the problem.

'At seven months, he still wasn't hearing any sounds, even with aids. Initially, we were against cochlear implants, as we didn't like the thought of him having major surgery.

'But, after his first birthday, with no response to any sounds, we realised it was what he would need to access the world of sound. We felt surprisingly calm as he went down to theatre, though it was awful seeing him so distressed when he came round from the anaesthetic. Within hours, though, he was calm and sleeping it off.

'We believe surgery was in Jamie's best interests but wouldn't judge anyone who didn't want it for their child. Just make sure you research the options thoroughly, and get the right information. We believe that some people who are against cochlear implants could tell you things which may not be true.

'We'd like him to attend a mainstream school, but we'll have to wait and see. Our hopes are really just the same as they would be for any hearing child – for him to try hard and do well and stay positive.'

'Before surgery, Jamie interacted well within the family but played alone. Now he plays with others kids. We go to a hearing playgroup every week and a monthly music group for deaf children, so he mixes with both groups. We hope he'll always have friends who can hear and those who can't.

'Since surgery, Jamie is happier and communicating much better. Implants have definitely changed all our lives for the better. He has an extremely good future with both hearing and speech if we work hard with him now. He recently told me he could hear birdsong. This is at a level of 20 to 30 decibels. Without the implant he could only hear at 125 decibels or above.

## Case Study

Helen's story

Helen, 52, is married to Mark and has two children. She now lives in Surrey but is originally from Kendal in the Lake District. With no hearing in her right ear, she has only 10% in her left.

Helen says: 'My hearing gradually got worse from the age of 14 onwards, when I was at grammar school. Note-taking was hard and my schoolwork quite messy. But I never wanted to admit to having a problem. When I was about 16, a doctor came to our house to look into it, but I wouldn't talk to him. I may have felt the whole thing was my fault.

'I started training as a nurse in Leeds in the 1970s, but never qualified. I was told I wasn't suitable. We worked on long wards and it was so hard to hear. There were no employment laws or rights back then and I was never taught to lipread. I did a secretarial course, had aids fitted and did a string of office jobs after that. But I had problems in nearly every one of my jobs – my employers just didn't understand what it was like to have a hearing problem.

'My son Nicholas was born in 1987, my daughter Rachel two years later. My hearing got worse after each pregnancy; it was so frustrating when I couldn't her what Rachel was saying, especially if she was in the middle of a tantrum! If she had friends round for tea, it was hard to hear them as well.

'I saw a hearing therapist and had a loop system fitted at home, but really I've never liked talking about my hearing difficulties to anyone.

'In May 2003, I was assessed for my suitability for a cochlear implant. This involved GP and speech therapist appointments, and visits to the ENT hospital in London. I also had tests to see how much I lipread.

'I had my cochlear implant fitted on my right side during a two-night stay in the ENT Hospital. I felt very groggy with severe headaches, but that didn't last. Six weeks later, it was tuned in. I had appointments every five or six weeks over the next two years or so, and the device was turned up to receive more intense sound each time.

'I just heard noise at first. It was as though my brain, not used to such loud volume, was trying to turn off what it could hear. But, now it's adjusted, I am able to enjoy music properly, especially if the song is one I remember from before my hearing got really bad. I can also have a conversation on the phone. My confidence has increased and I don't tire quite so easily.

'An implant is very different from a hearing aid, in that it channels speech and helps the brain to block out sounds which it doesn't need.

'It's only after the operation that I've come to realise just how bad my hearing was before. I now visit people who are considering implants as a volunteer, to reassure them. The hospital has regular get-togethers for its cochlear implant patients, so I get support that way as well.

'My cochlear implant has given me my life back. I can feel part of living again without the isolation and loneliness that lack of communication brings.'

'My cochlear implant has given me my life back. I can feel part of living again without the isolation and loneliness that lack of communication brings.'

# Summing Up

■ A cochlear implant is a device which works through direct electrical stimulation of the auditory nerve.

■ It is not a 'miracle cure'.

■ Those who are most likely to benefit include those who were born deaf or adults who had speech before losing their hearing.

■ There are two parts to cochlear implants – an externally worn processor and the implant itself, surgically inserted beneath the skull during major, invasive irreversible surgery.

■ Processors can be worn on the body or behind the ear.

■ You must undergo a thorough assessment for your suitability for an implant before surgery can go ahead.

■ Traditionally there has been resistance to cochlear implantation from some members of the Deaf community, who see themselves as part of a cultural minority rather than as having a medical problem.

# Chapter Ten

# Living with Hearing Loss

## Older people and hearing loss

### The facts

As we saw in chapter 1, ageing is the single most common factor behind all deafness and hearing loss.

In the UK, approaching three quarters of those over 70 will have some kind of hearing loss. Just over a quarter of these will experience mild loss, around 36% a moderate loss, 6.3% a severe loss and 1.3% a profound hearing loss.

For those aged over 50, the figures are as follows:

- Nearly 42% will have some kind of hearing loss.

- Just over a fifth will have a mild hearing loss.

- For moderate and severe hearing loss, the figures are 16.8% and 2.7% respectively.

- 0.6% of over 50-year-olds will have profound hearing loss

(Source: RNID.)

While hearing loss and deafness and their severity are different in every individual, there is a pattern to age-related hearing loss. The hair cells which pick up high frequency sounds are usually damaged first. The severity of the loss differs in each case, but often the low frequencies will be less affected, so you get a typical 'ski-slope' loss. Some people's hearing will gradually

'While hearing loss and deafness and their severity are different in every individual, there is a pattern to age-related hearing loss.'

deteriorate over time and will begin to affect the low frequencies too. Other people's hearing loss remains quite stable and little change is seen in the pattern of hearing loss over time

## Older people and hearing aids

It can be difficult to adjust to hearing aids at any age, but so much depends on how long you leave a hearing loss without doing somthing about it. People often wait until they have had a hearing loss for quite a long while before seeking help. Over this time, their hearing will have gradually deteriorated and they will not have been hearing certain sounds for some time. This can make it harder to adapt to the sound of the hearing aid as the brain needs to learn how to process these sounds again.

While people of any age may be reluctant to start using a hearing aid, in older people dexterity can be a problem, particularly if someone has arthritis or does not have much feeling in their fingers. However, digital hearing aids can be programmed to automatically adjust to sounds, giving priority to speech. So, once in the ear, you don't have to fiddle with them unless you want to use the loop system, which is set up on a different programme. Volume control can also be set up to adjust automatically.

As we saw in chapter 7, it is always worth trying lipreading classes as this is a great way to support hearing aid use. Lipreading classes can help you to make the best use of the hearing you have and to communicate better by developing your lipreading and observational skills.

This can be particularly important for older people, for whom isolation as a result of their hearing loss can be an issue.

# Living with someone with a hearing loss

## How to tell someone may be losing their hearing

- You may find that your parent or partner needs much of the conversation repeated several times, or misunderstands what is being said.

- They may complain that you are not speaking clearly or loudly enough.

- They may seem anxious in situations which were previously not worrying, or don't take pleasure from social events which they previously enjoyed.

- They may not hear you when you enter the room.

- They may not hear the phone or doorbell.

- They may struggle with pubs, parties and other noisy environments.

- They may turn the television or radio up so loudly that the volume is uncomfortable.

- Speech may have become a monotone and less clear than it used to be.

- You may find they talk more than they used to, since speaking has become less of a strain than listening.

With gradual hearing loss, high frequency sounds which carry consonants tend to be lost first and lipreading becomes relied on more and more to fill in the gaps (see chapter 7 for more about lipreading).

## Seeking help

Whatever age someone close to you starts to experience deafness or hearing loss, they should seek help as soon as they are able to. Encourage them to do this.

It's better to find out about hearing aids and start wearing them sooner rather than later, since getting used to amplified sound can be harder if the person has already grown used to a 'quieter' world.

You could also suggest they try RNID's hearing check – this assesses your ability to hear someone speaking when there's background noise. You can take the test on their website or over the telephone on 0844 800 3838. The test takes about five minutes.

'It is important that you understand what has happened to your parent or partner's hearing. You both need to accept the hearing loss and be positive about it.'

## How can I help someone close to me?

It is important that you understand what has happened to your parent or partner's hearing. You both need to accept the hearing loss and be positive about it.

- Be supportive and patient and accept that sometimes there will be frustrations.

- Don't try and do everything – if the doorbell rings, for example, encourage them to answer it.

- Try not to either speak for them or exclude them from the conversation.

- Encourage them to discuss their hearing loss with friends and other family members.

- Don't think their deafness or hearing loss has to mean an end to your own regular social activities, or that you can't sometimes do the things you enjoy on your own.

- Don't let your parent/partner apologise for their hearing impairment – it is no one's fault. Equally, oddly, sometimes other people will apologise for someone being deaf. Try to discourage this.

- Set a good example to others by speaking clearly and a little more slowly, but without shouting, so you can be understood. This should give others a better idea of what to do.

- Encourage your parent/partner to ask their GP to examine their ears as soon as problems start. The GP may refer your parent/partner to a specialist at an ENT unit in the hospital or directly to the audiology department. Because NHS waiting lists can be long, you should start the process as soon as possible.

- Walk on the deaf person's 'better' side if appropriate.

- Hearing loss does not have to affect your relationship with someone – in many ways you do not have to treat them any differently to the way you did before they started to lose their hearing.

## What will we have to cope with?

- Just chatting becomes hard work and can be tiring.

- Both not hearing and having to repeat things can be exasperating – sometimes the temptation to say 'it doesn't matter' can be overwhelming.

- The person you are close to may become irritable because they are frustrated, or they become very withdrawn.

- Your family member will have less time to relax because they will be focusing more on communicating.

- A deaf or hearing impaired person may find that they cannot hear their own voice, so they don't realise how loud their speech is for others. Also, some hard of hearing people may slur some of their speech sounds because they cannot hear their own voice to correct themselves.

- Wearing a hearing aid for the first time can seem a huge step. Encourage use as much as possible and for it to be worn as visibly as possible, so others know there is a problem. If the aid doesn't appear to be working properly, encourage a return to the specialist who fitted it. If possible, you should go along as well, so you can understand how it works and how to maintain and look after it.

- If your parent/partner loses their hearing, you may have to deal with more of the things that maybe they used to sort out, such as holiday or restaurant bookings, or talking to the bank or electricity company.

## What about me?

Of course, deafness can be stressful and frustrating at times, both for the person experiencing it and for anyone who is close to them. If you live with someone who has a hearing loss, either as a parent, partner, son or daughter, it's important to both acknowledge the fact and take care of yourself as well. Make sure you have a relative, friend or someone else you can talk to, and who can lighten the load.

Be open with the person who has the loss. Let them know how you are feeling, rather than bottling up your frustrations.

# Benefits and pensions

Your hearing loss may entitle you, or someone you live with, to some state benefits.

The Department for Work and Pensions (DWP) assesses and pays benefits in England, Wales and Scotland. If you live in Northern Ireland, contact the Benefit Enquiry Line for Northern Ireland for more advice.

## Attendance Allowance (AA)

**'If you are either registered deaf or the user of an NHS hearing aid or in receipt of a benefit such as Attendance Allowance, you can apply for a Disabled Person's Railcard.'**

If you are over 65 and have a disability which has an impact on your daily life or means you need extra help to communicate every day, you may be entitled to claim this allowance. This is not a means-tested benefit, and you don't have to be paying National Insurance contributions to qualify.

## Disability Living Allowance (DLA)

This benefit is for children and adults up to the age of 64, whether they are studying, in work or not working. It is not taxable or means-tested, and it's non-contributory, meaning you can be eligible even if you don't pay National Insurance contributions. If you are making a claim, do so sooner rather than later, since claims cannot usually be back-dated.

There are two elements to DLA – a care component and a mobility component. You may be eligible for both or either of these elements, but you need to pass certain disability tests first.

Contact your local social security or Jobcentre Plus office, visit the DWP website or call the Benefit Enquiry Line for more information (see help list for details).

## Disabled Person's Railcard

If you are either registered deaf or the user of an NHS hearing aid or in receipt of a benefit such as Attendance Allowance, you can apply for one of these railcards. Priced at £18 for a year or £48 for three years (at the time of going to press), this card allows you a third off most UK rail fares. The great advantage it has over other concessionary fares, such as Network Railcards, is that you can take someone with you and they will get the same discount. Equally, you can use this railcard all the time, not just at off-peak times. Pick up a leaflet from your local station or visit www.disabledpersonsrailcard.co.uk.

## Industrial Injuries Disablement Benefit

If you have become deafened by noise at work over time (occupational deafness) or following an accident in your job, you may qualify for this benefit. It is non-contributory or means-tested and you can still claim if you are working now.

To claim occupational deafness, you need to have been working as a salaried employee in one of the DWP's listed occupations for at least 10 years and you must have been in this job within the last five years of the date you first make your claim. The level of your loss will be assessed during a hearing test.

## Armed service

If your hearing was affected while serving in the armed forces, you may be entitled to War Disablement Pension or Armed Forces Compensation, which replaces the War Pensions Scheme for anyone made deaf or disabled while serving on or after April 2005. There are strict rules in place for claiming these benefits. If you were disabled as a civilian during wartime, you may also qualify. Visit www.veterans-uk.info for more information.

## Carer's Allowance

Those caring for someone who receives Attendance Allowance, or sometimes Disability Living Allowance, may be able to claim this benefit.

## Pension Credit

This means-tested benefit is for those over 60, and there are two parts to it. Contact your local pension service, who will visit you at home and advise you how to go about claiming a wide range of benefits.

## Case study

Michael, 53, from the South West, first started to lose his hearing more than 20 years ago. He has written a book about his experiences with his hearing dog, Matt, called *If It Wasn't For that Dog*.

He says: 'A GP read from the newspaper to see what I could hear and I had a hearing test. I found I only had 25% hearing in my left ear and 40% in my right. I had a genetic condition called accelerated degradation of hair cells in the cochlea. We all have a given number of hair cells to start with and they tend to drop off with age. I started with fewer than other people and mine were just wearing out much more quickly.

'They fitted a hearing aid, but I didn't really understand what was going on, there didn't seem to be any personal back up. I was married at the time, with two young daughters who didn't quite understand what was happening. I admit I became quite reclusive and difficult to live with.

'In 2001, my wife left and so I had to deal with that. A breakthrough came when I started going to a lipreading class in New Milton every week. I learned about the help which was available and realised I wasn't alone. At around the same time, I joined a local creative writing group which gave me another new lease of life. I met Jacquie, who also has a hearing loss and who also loves writing. She is now my partner.

'In 2004, I was given my hearing dog Matt after being interviewed by Hearing Dogs for the Deaf and put on their waiting list. I fell in love with him from the moment I first saw a picture of him! He was trained for a year, and that included the sound work and obedience training.

'Matt can hear the doorbell, smoke alarm, phone and the fire alarm where I work. He acts as my alarm clock every morning. If necessary, he can alert me to danger by lying flat on the floor. All this is, of course, very helpful, but it's just as important that he makes the invisible problem of hearing visible. People want to know about him as I walk around the supermarket and so on. He is a real talking point. I've learned to stand my ground in restaurants and places where people try to ban him as he's legally entitled to entry.'

Need2Know

# Summing Up

■ Hearing loss is almost an inevitable aspect of growing older. Hearing cells which pick up the high frequency sounds are usually the first to be damaged.

■ Older people can find it hard to insert and remove hearing aids because their fingers may not be so nimble.

■ If you think you or someone close to you are losing hearing, take action as soon as possible. The longer the problem is left, the worse things become.

■ There are many things you can do to help and support someone close to you who has a hearing loss.

■ If you live with someone who loses their hearing, it can affect your life too. Make sure your needs are not forgotten about.

■ Deaf and hard of hearing people are entitled to a range of benefits and pension credits. Make sure you claim everything to which you are entitled.

# Help List

## Access to Work

www.direct.gov.uk
Government scheme providing employers advice and support with extra costs which may arise because of your needs. Click on 'disabled people' then 'work schemes and programmes' to find the Access to Work scheme.

## Association of Teachers of Lipreading to Adults (ATLA)

c/o Hearing Concern LINK, 19 Hartfield Road, Eastbourne, E. Sussex, BN21 2AR
atla@lipreading.org.uk
www.lipreading.org.uk
Membership association for qualified teachers of lipreading, not open to the general public, but can help you find lipreading classes in your area.

## Benefit Enquiry Line (NI)

Tel: 0800 220 674 (helpline)
www.dsdni.gov.uk
Provides general advice and information for disabled people and carers on the range of benefits available.

## Benefit Enquiry Line (UK)

Red Rose House, Lancaster Road, Preston, Lancashire, PR1 1HB
Tel: 0800 882 200 (helpline, Monday to Friday, 8.30am-6.30pm, Saturday 9am-1pm)
BEL-Customer-Services@dwp.gsi.gov.uk
www.direct.gov.uk/disability-money
Provides general advice and information for disabled people and carers on the range of benefits available.

# British Cochlear Implant Group

www.bcig.org.uk

National organisation promoting benefits of cochlear implants for children and adults. Regional contact details can be found in the 'contact us' section of the website.

# British Deaf Association

10th Floor, Coventry Point, Market Way, Coventry, CV1 1EA

Tel: 02476 550936

headoffice@bda.org.uk

www.bda.org.uk

The BDA is the largest Deaf organisation in the UK run by Deaf people. It represents the sign language community.

# British-Sign

Honeysuckle Cottage, Les Dunes, Vazon, Castel, Guernsey, GY5 7LQ

Tel: 02071 173829

info@british-sign.co.uk

www.british-sign.co.uk

Commercial organisation providing online British Sign Language courses.

# British Tinnitus Association

Ground Floor, Unit 5, Acorn Business Park, Woodseats Close, Sheffield, S8 0TB

Tel: 0800 018 0527 (helpline, Monday to Friday, 9am-5pm)

info@tinnitus.org.uk

www.tinnitus.org.uk

National organisation providing information and support about tinnitus for those who have tinnitus and the medical professionals who work with them.

# Chambers and Partners

Saville House, 23 Long Lane, London, EC1A 9HL

Tel: 020 7606 8844

www.chambersandpartners.com

Publisher of the world's leading guides on the legal profession. To search for a lawyer in your area just search under the name of your nearest city.

## Deafblind UK

John and Lucille van Geest Place, Cygnet Road, Hampton, Peterborough, PE7 8FD
Tel: 0800 132 320 (information line)
Info@deafblind.org.uk
www.deafblind.org.uk
National charity supporting people with a combined sight and hearing loss.

## Deafness Research UK (The Hearing Research Trust)

330-332 Gray's Inn Road, London, WC1X 8EE
Tel: 0808 808 2222 (helpline, Monday to Friday, 9am-5pm)
contact@deafnessresearch.org.uk
www.deafnessresearch.org.uk
Medical charity for deaf and hard of hearing people, working to improve the prevention, diagnosis and treatment of all forms of hearing impairment.

## Department for Children, Schools and Families (DCSF)

Castle View House, East Lane, Runcorn, Cheshire, WA7 2GJ
Tel: 0870 000 2288
www.dcsf.gov.uk
Government department leading a network of people who work with or for children and young people.

## Department for Work and Pensions (DWP)

www.dwp.gov.uk
Government department responsible for welfare and pension reform. Click on 'contact us' for your local office search or an A-Z of helpline numbers.

## Direct Gov

www.direct.gov.uk
Government website where all public services are listed and some information and contact details can be found on each.

## Disability Law Service

39-45 Cavell Street, London, E1 2BP
Tel: 020 7791 9800
advice@dls.org.uk
www.dls.org.uk
Provides high quality information and advice to disabled and Deaf people.

## Disabled Persons Railcard

Rail Travel Made Easy, PO Box 11631, Laurencekirk, AB30 9AA
Tel: 0845 605 0525
disability@atoc.org
www.disabledpersons-railcard.co.uk
If you have a disability which makes travelling difficult, you get a third off most rail fares in the UK.

## The Ear Foundation

Marjorie Sherman House, 83 Sherwin Road, Lenton, Nottingham, NG7 2FB
Tel: 0115 942 1985
www.earfoundation.org.uk
Provides independent information, training and support for deaf children and young adults with cochlear implants, their families and professionals.

## Hearing Aid Council

70 St Mary Axe, London, EC3A 8BE
Tel: 020 3102 4030
hac@thehearingaidcouncil.org.uk
www.thehearingaidcouncil.org.uk
The government body which sets standards in the private hearing aid market.

## Hearing Concern LINK

19 Hartfield Road , Eastbourne, East Sussex, BN21 2AR
Tel: 01323 638230
info@hearingconcernlink.org
www.hearingconcernlink.org

Charity providing support and information to those with a hearing loss and their families (formerly two separate charities, Hearing Concern and the LINK Centre for Deafened People).

## Hearing Dogs for Deaf People

The Grange, Wycombe Road, Saunderton, Princes Risborough, Buckinghamshire, HP27 9NS
Tel: 01844 348 100
info@hearingdogs.org.uk
www.hearingdogs.org.uk
National organisation which works to help deaf and hard of hearing people through the training and placement of specially trained dogs.

## Jobcentre Plus

www.jobcentreplus.gov.uk
You can report a change in circumstances for your benefits and find information on getting back to work.

## Law Society

www.lawsociety.org.uk
This website is a starting point if you are looking for an employment lawyer.

## National Association of Deafened People

PO Box 50, Amersham, HP6 6XB
Tel: 0845 055 9663
enquiries@nadp.org.uk
www.nadp.org.uk
National organisation offering support for deafened people who have lost all or most of their useful hearing, either gradually or suddenly, their families and friends.

## National Deaf Children's Society (NDCS)

15 Dufferin Street, London, EC1Y 8UR
Tel: 0808 800 8880 (helpline, Monday to Friday, 9.30am-5pm, Saturday 9.30am-12pm)
ndcs@ndcs.org.uk
www.ndcs.org.uk

National organisation working to support all deaf children and young people, their families and the professional working with them.

## National Institute for Clinical Excellence (NICE)

MidCity Place, 71 High Holborn, London, WC1V 6NA
Tel: 0845 003 7780
nice@nice.org.uk
www.nice.org.uk
Independent organisation responsible for providing national guidance on the promotion of good health and the prevention and treatment of ill health.

## NHS Newborn Screening Programme

www.hearing.screening.nhs.uk
Government run screening programme to ensure all parents are offered hearing screening for their new child within the first few weeks of life.

## Ofcom

Riverside House, 2a Southwark Bridge Road, London, SE1 9HA
Tel: 0300 123 3000 or 020 7981 3000
www.ofcom.org.uk
Ofcom regulates TV and radio, fixed line telecoms and mobiles and the airwaves over which wireless devices operate and is responsible for the regulation of television access service (subtitling, signing and audio description).

## Peltor

www.peltor.com
Manufacturer of ear muffs and defenders.

## Quality Assurance Agency for Higher Education (QAA)

Southgate House, Southgate Street, Gloucester, GL1 1UB
Tel: 01452 557000
comms@qaa.ac.uk
www.qaa.ac.uk
Responsible for safeguarding quality and standards in UK higher education.

## RNID

19-23 Featherstone Street, London, EC1Y 8SL
Tel: 0808 808 0123 (information line)
informationline@rnid.org.uk
www.rnid.org.uk
RNID is the charity working to create a world where deafness or hearing loss
do not limit or determine opportunity, and where people value their hearing.
It works by campaigning and lobbying, raising awareness of deafness and
hearing loss, promoting hearing health, providing services and through social,
medical and technical research.

## SENDIST

Mowden Hall, Staindrop Road, DL3 9BG
Tel: 01325 392760
www.sendist.gov.uk
The independent body which considers cases where LAs and parents cannot
agree on the special educational needs of a child.

## Teachernet

www.teachernet.gov.uk
Website with information regarding special educational needs.

## Veterans UK

www.veterans-uk.info
Veterans UK is the single point of contact for accessing information on war
disablement pension or armed forces compensation.

# References

Bamford, J, Fortnum, H, Bristow, K, Smith, J, Vamvakas, G, Davies, L, Taylor, R, Watkin P, Fonseca, S and Hind, S (2007) 'Current practice, accuracy, effectiveness and cost-effectiveness of the school entry hearing screen', *Health Technology Assessment*, vol. 11, issue 32, pages 1-188.

Fortnum, H, Summerfield, A, Marshall, D, Davis, A and Bamford, J (2001) 'Prevalence of permanent childhood hearing impairment in the United Kingdom and implications for universal neonatal hearing screening: questionnaire based ascertainment study', *BMJ*, vol. 323, page 536.

NDCS (2008) *Living with a deaf child, a sibling perspective*. Unpublished.

Rawlings, BW and Jensema, CJ (1977) *Two studies of the families of hearing impaired children*, Washington, DC: Gallaudet College Office of Demographic Studies.

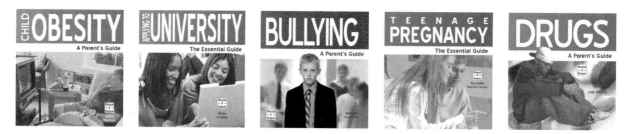